the DIABETES
recipe book

Bounty
Books

The Diabetes Recipe Book

Publisher: Samantha Warrington
Managing Editor: Karen Rigden
Production Controller: Sarah Kramer
Editor: Jane Birch
Designer: Chris Bell/cbdesign

Published in 2015 by Bounty Books,
a division of Octopus Publishing Group Ltd
Carmelite House
50 Victoria Embankment
London, EC4Y 0DZ
www.octopusbooks.co.uk

An Hachette UK Company
www.hachette.co.uk

ISBN: 978-0-753729-29-8

Printed and bound in China

contents

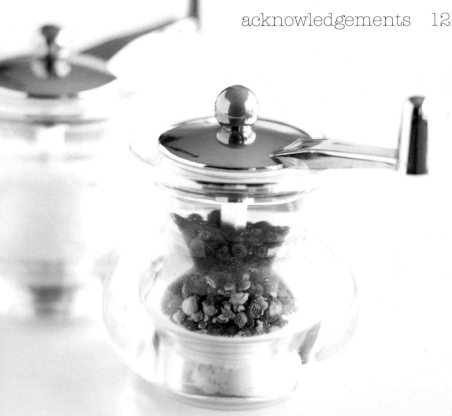

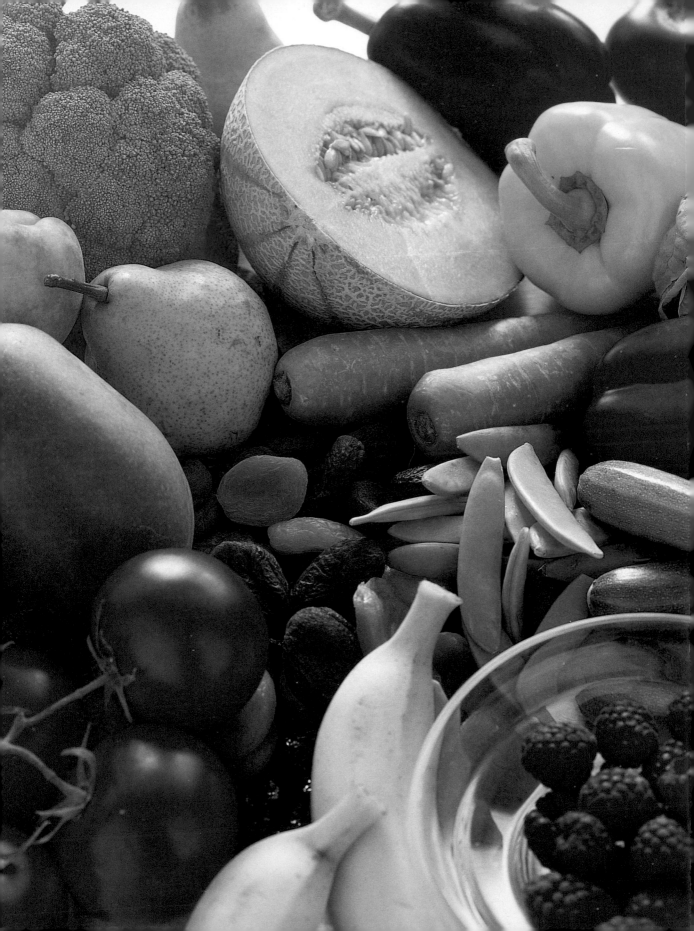

introduction

What is diabetes?

Diabetes is a common condition in which the glucose (sugar) level in the blood is too high. Normally, the level of glucose in the blood is controlled by a hormone called insulin, which is produced in the pancreas. Insulin enables the glucose to enter various cells in the body, where it is used to fuel the body's energy requirements. When you have diabetes, the body doesn't produce any or enough insulin to regulate the glucose, or the insulin that it does produce does not do the job properly. As a result, the glucose is unable to get into the cells where it is needed to provide energy and, instead, remains in the blood stream at high levels.

There are two main types of diabetes:

Type 1 or insulin dependent diabetes This develops when the body stops producing insulin because the cells in the pancreas that make it have been destroyed. It usually appears before the age of 40 and is treated by insulin injections and diet.

Type 2 or non-insulin dependent diabetes This is the most common type of diabetes. It develops when the body can still produce insulin, but not enough for its needs or when the insulin that it does produce does not work properly. It usually appears in people over the age of 40 and may be treated by diet alone, or by diet in conjunction with tablets or insulin injections. People who are overweight are more likely to develop Type 2 diabetes and around 80 per cent of people who are diagnosed with Type 2 are overweight.

Nutrition and diabetes

If you are diagnosed with diabetes, you should aim to shift the balance of your diet to control your blood glucose levels and to help you manage your condition more easily.

Start by assessing your current eating habits and consider any changes that you need to make. You should consider your food choices or meal planning in the context of a framework, rather than as rigid rules that can never be broken. Establishing long-term healthy eating habits can also help you reach other targets, such as your ideal weight and good cholesterol and blood pressure levels.

Diabetes fact
It is estimated that 300 million people worldwide will have diabetes by 2025.

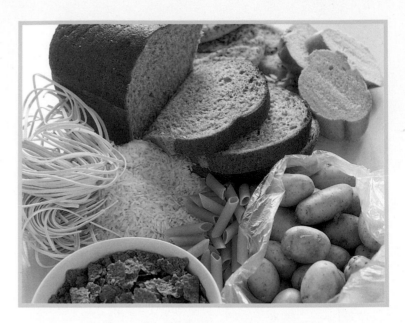

The nutritional goals you set yourself do not have to seem impossible; they can be as simple and straightforward as snacking on a piece of fruit, rather than a biscuit, or adding an extra portion of salad or vegetables to your evening meal.

Many people still believe that, if you have diabetes, you have to stick to a rigid diet and cut out foods such as cakes and desserts. This is not the case at all and, whatever your individual dietary needs, the meals you make for yourself can still be delicious and just as suitable for family and friends to enjoy. As long as you get it right most of the time, you can also enjoy treats and special-occasion meals. You'll find some delicious recipes for food to share with friends on pages 84–109, plus recipes for desserts on pages 110–125.

Seeing a dietitian

Anyone diagnosed with diabetes should be referred to a registered dietitian through their doctor or hospital. A dietitian will provide specific dietary advice and help you work out targets based on your particular needs and lifestyle, which will help you to feel more in control of your diabetes.

Healthy eating guidelines

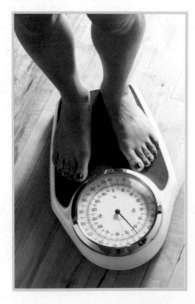

Watch your weight This is an essential aspect of diabetes care. Being overweight makes it difficult to control blood glucose levels, cholesterol levels and blood pressure. So it is important to try to get to the weight that is right for you and to stay there. If you need to lose weight, aim for a gradual weight loss that you can maintain in the long term.

Have regular meals Eat regularly throughout the day and base your meals on starchy carbohydrates such as bread, potatoes, rice, pasta and cereals. Go one step better and opt for carbs with a low GI (glycaemic index) rating, such as wholemeal pasta, wholegrain cereals, fruit and pulses. (See page 10 for more about GI.)

Cut down on saturated fat Aim to cut down on foods that are rich in saturated fat, such as fatty meats, butter, cheese and cream. Instead, opt for low-fat spreads high in unsaturated fat (olive, rapeseed or sunflower oil) and substitute low-fat natural yogurt, crème fraîche or fromage frais for cream. Swap creamy sauces for tomato-based ones instead. Eat fats that are good for you, including olive oil, nuts and avocados.

There are a some simple ways to cut down on fat when cooking:
• Grill, bake, poach or steam rather than frying or roasting.
• Use lean cuts of meat and poultry and remove visible fat and skin before cooking.
• Skim fat off after cooking.

Cut down on salt Try not to add salt to your food. Experiment with flavourings like herbs, spices and lemon or lime juice. Look out for reduced-salt bread, canned foods, stock and sauces to add to your shopping basket. Also, be aware of overdoing the salty snacks, such as crisps and nuts.

Eat more fruit, vegetable and pulses
To balance your meals and get a wide range of antioxidant vitamins and minerals, you should try to eat five portions of fruit, veg and pulses a day. See the box opposite for some guidelines about what counts as a portion.

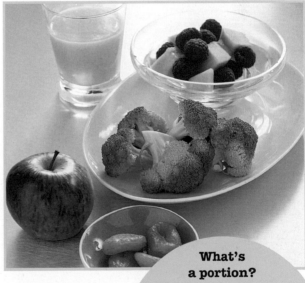

Limit your intake of sugary food and drink Your diet doesn't have to be sugar free but try to avoid sweet treats like chocolate, cake and fizzy drinks, especially if you are trying to lose weight. Save them for special occasions and you'll enjoy them all the more.

Keep alcohol to safe limits This means a maximum of two units per day (which is equal to one small glass of wine, one measure of spirits or half a pint of beer) for women and three units per day for men. Never drink on an empty stomach.

What's a portion?
One portion = a piece of fruit, such as a banana or apple, a handful of grapes, a small glass of fruit juice or smoothie, three heaped tablespoons of vegetables, a small bowl of salad.

Simple swaps for better nutrition

Instead of...	try
White rice	Brown, wild or basmati rice
Potatoes	Sweet potato, butternut squash, yam
White pasta	Wholemeal pasta
White bread	Wholewheat and granary bread
Instant porridge	Rolled oats
Cornflakes	Bran flakes
Sugary cereal	Natural muesli
Cream	Low fat crème fraîche or yogurt
Full-fat milk	Semi-skimmed or skimmed milk
Frying or roasting	Grilling, steaming, oven-baking

Diabetes tip
Packed with minerals, vitamins and fibre, fruit is a great way to satisfy a sweet tooth. End a meal with a fresh fruit salad or choose fruit as a healthy snack.

Understanding GI

All carbohydrate foods are reduced to glucose when they are digested, but at different rates and in varying amounts. The glycaemic index (GI) is a ranking – from 0 to 100 – of carbohydrate-containing foods based on the overall effect on blood glucose levels.

For example, mashed potato has a rating of 70 which is high, compared to boiled sweet potato which, at 54, is low. White rice has a high GI rating of 87 compared to medium GI basmati rice which rates at 58.

Slowly absorbed foods have a low GI rating, while foods that are more quickly absorbed have a higher rating. This is important because choosing slowly absorbed carbohydrates, instead of quickly absorbed carbohydrates, is a useful way to help you manage your diabetes.

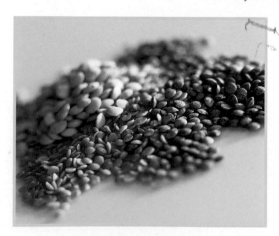

Choosing lower GI foods can help you to maintain your blood glucose levels, minimizing fluctuations. Low GI foods can also help to control appetite by making you feel fuller for longer, so that you eat less. While it important to try to eat lower GI foods on a regular basis if you can, remember it is not about cutting out high GI foods altogether. Instead, aim for a balanced diet.

To reduce the overall GI of your diet, you can incorporate more starchy carbs with a low GI, such as bulgar wheat, pearl barley, wholewheat pasta, rye bread, pumpernickel bread, basmati rice, sweet potatoes, oats, pulses and lentils.

The perfect plate

Your overall daily diet should aim to include the right proportions of the main food groups:

1 Starchy carbohydrates These should form the largest portion of your diet. You should base meals and snacks around these foods when possible.

2 Fruit and vegetables Fruit and veg should make the second largest portion of your daily diet. Aim to get at least five portions per day.

3 Milk and dairy foods These should make up the third largest portion of your diet. Choose low-fat dairy foods and spreads where you can.

4 Meat, fish and other protein foods Choose lean meat and poultry, fish, pulses or other protein foods. They should form the second smallest portion of your diet.

5 Fats, oils and sugary foods These should be the smallest portion of your daily diet. Avoid fatty and sugary foods wherever possible, indulging only occasionally.

Diabetes and exercise

Alongside healthier eating habit, getting moving is vital. Exercise is good for all of us. Among its many benefits, it boosts mental health, cuts the risk of stress and depression, helps you lose or maintain weight, boosts the immune system and cuts the risk of cardiovascular disease. For people with diabetes being active helps the body use insulin more efficiently and gives you better blood sugar control.

According to government health guidelines, we should all be aiming for 150 minutes of moderate intensity aerobic exercise – such as fast walking, light jogging, swimming, rowing or tennis – a week.

Get the whole family to join you or ask a friend to be your exercise buddy, so that you can combine socializing with being fit. Be it badminton, karate or zumba, finding an activity you enjoy means you are more likely to stick with your exercise plan.

Living with diabetes

If you have diabetes you will inevitably have to make some changes to your way of life. But, simply by thinking more about what you eat and how you shop for and cook food, you should be able to continue your normal life. Having diabetes doesn't mean having to go without life's pleasures, it simply means that you need to make some healthier choices.

Go for a walk
Ideal for all ages and fitness levels, regular walking reduces the risk of chronic illnesses such as heart disease, asthma, stroke and some cancers.

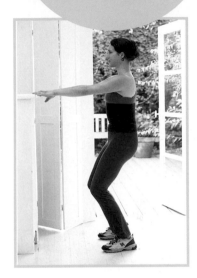

Your healthy habits checklist

- Choose wholegrain pasta, bread and cereals
- Eat lots of fruit and veg
- Cut down on saturated fat
- Choose 'good' fat
- Eat lean meat
- Eat more fish
- Avoid sugary drinks
- Exercise daily
- Drink alcohol in moderation
- Watch portion sizes
- Have regular meals
- Cut down on salt

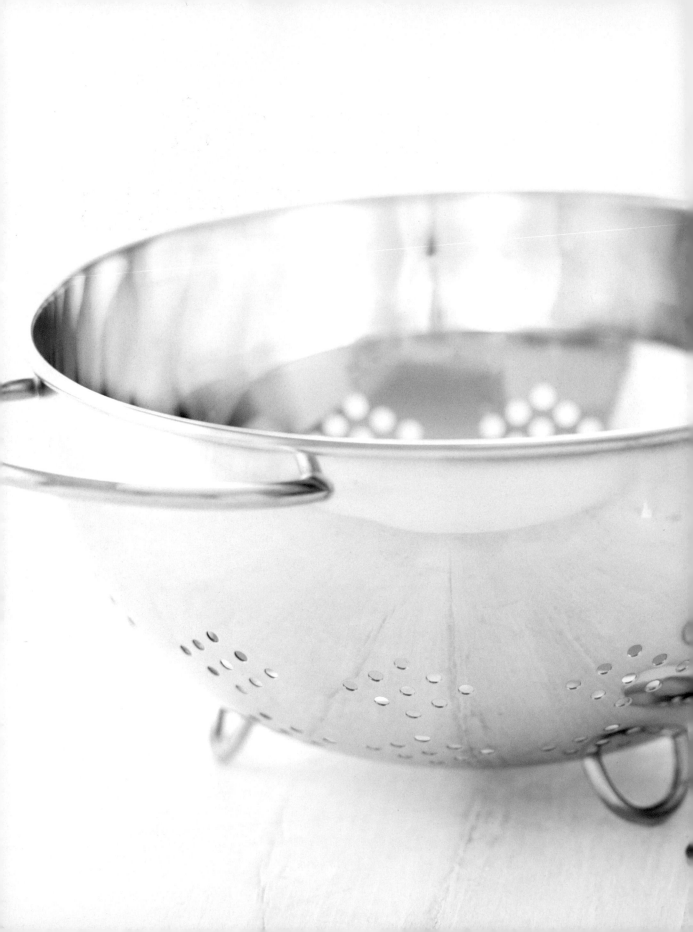

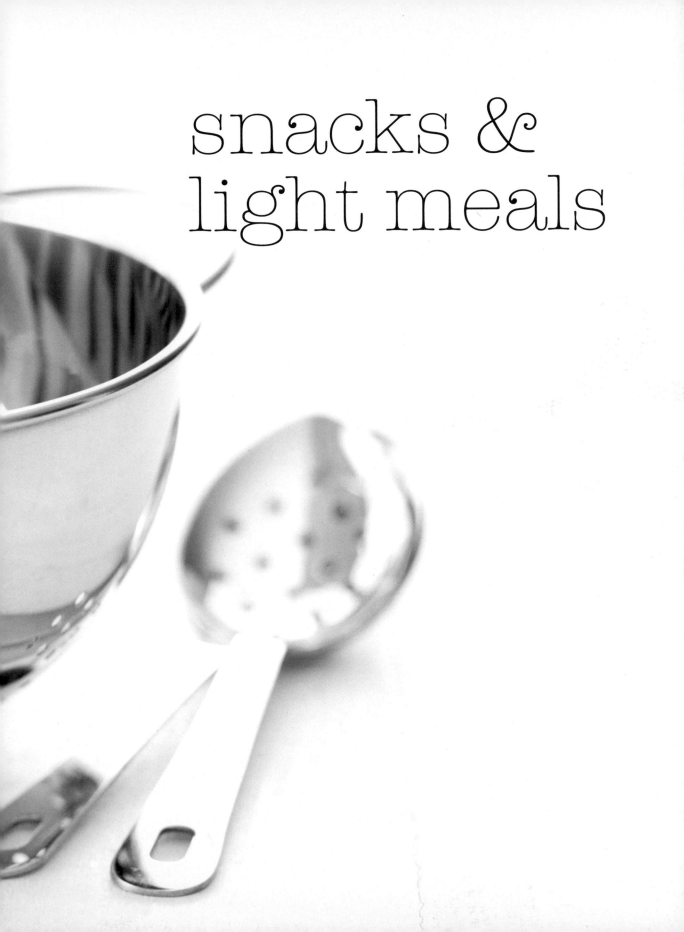

snacks &
light meals

guacamole

serves 4
prep + cook time 10 minutes

2 ripe avocados, peeled, stoned
   and chopped
juice of 1 lime
6 cherry tomatoes, diced
1 tablespoon chopped coriander
1–2 garlic cloves, crushed
oatcakes or vegetable crudités,
   to serve

1 Put the avocados and lime juice in a bowl and mash together
to prevent discoloration, then stir in the remaining ingredients.
2 Serve immediately with oatcakes or vegetable crudités.

Tip
Although high
in calories, avocados
pack a mighty nutritional
punch with nearly
20 vitamins and minerals
and are a rich source of
monounsaturated
'good' fat.

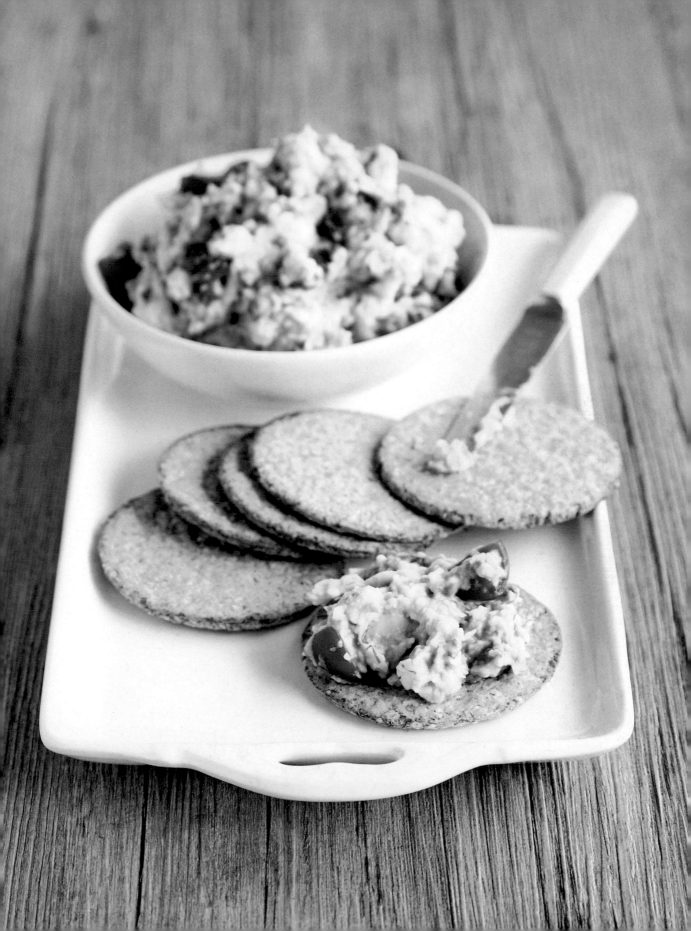

spring onion & potato pasties

makes 12
prep + cook time 30–35 minutes

375 g (12 oz) ready-made
   shortcrust pastry
plain flour, for dusting
a little milk, for brushing

filling
1 medium potato, cut into small
   cubes
4 spring onions, sliced
45 g (1¾ oz) sweetcorn kernels,
   defrosted if frozen
2 tablespoons reduced-fat crème
   fraîche
salt and pepper

1 Roll out the pastry on a lightly floured work surface to a thickness of 3 mm (⅛ inch). Using a saucer, cut out 12 rounds of pastry, 12 cm (5 inches) in diameter.
2 Cook the potatoes in a pan of boiling water for 5 minutes, then drain. Mix with the spring onions, sweetcorn and crème fraîche and season to taste with salt and pepper. Place a little of the mixture to one side of the centre of each piece of pastry.
3 Dampen the edges of the pastry with a little water and fold in half to cover the filling.
4 Press down the edges with a fork, then place on a greased baking sheet. Brush with a little milk, then cook in a preheated oven at 200°C (400°F), Gas Mark 6 for 15–20 minutes until golden brown.

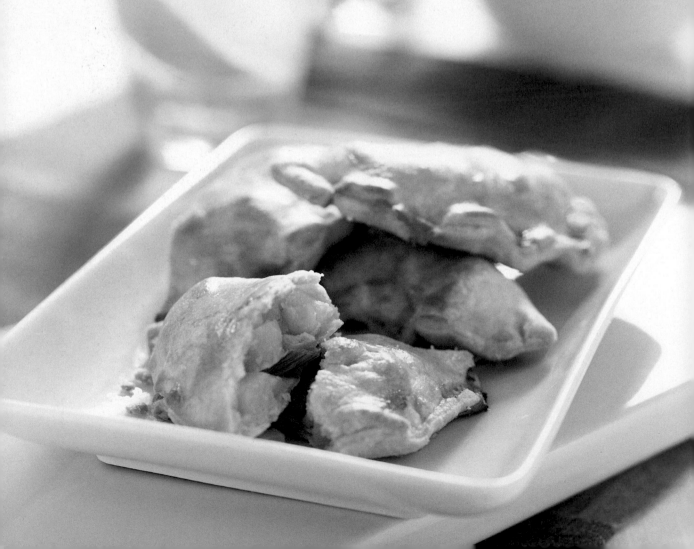

herby bean cakes

serves 4
prep + cook time 25 minutes

2 x 400 g (13 oz) cans cannellini
   beans, drained and rinsed
2 eggs, beaten
1 bunch of spring onions, finely
   chopped
4 tablespoons chopped herbs,
   such as sage, parsley or thyme
50 g (2 oz) Stilton cheese,
   crumbled
4 tablespoons plain flour
50 g (2 oz) fine white breadcrumbs
2 tablespoons oil
salt and pepper
4 parsley sprigs, to garnish
tomato and cucumber salad,
   to serve

1 Place the beans in a food processor or blender and blend until almost smooth. Add half of the egg and blend again.
2 Stir in the spring onions, herbs and Stilton. Season to taste with salt and pepper.
3 Shape the mixture into 8 balls, then flatten them slightly with the palm of your hand. Coat the patties in flour, then dip them into the remaining egg, then in the breadcrumbs, to coat them. Place on a lightly oiled baking sheet and drizzle with the oil.
4 Cook the bean cakes in a preheated oven at 200°C (400°F), Gas Mark 6 for 10–15 minutes until golden and piping hot. Garnish each serving with a parsley sprig and serve with a tomato and cucumber salad.

Tip
Fresh parsley is
a good source of
vitamin C and iron.

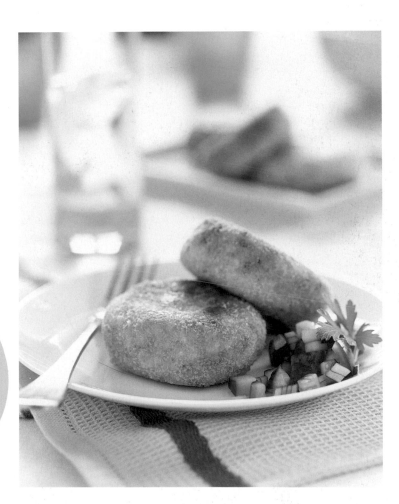

chicken burgers with tomato salsa

serves 4
prep + cook time 25 minutes + chilling time

1 garlic clove, crushed
3 spring onions, finely sliced
1 tablespoon pesto
2 tablespoons chopped mixed
    herbs, such as parsley, tarragon
    and thyme
375 g (12 oz) minced chicken
2 sun-dried tomatoes, finely
    chopped
1 teaspoon olive oil

tomato salsa
250 g (8 oz) cherry tomatoes,
    quartered
1 red chilli, deseeded and finely
    chopped
1 tablespoon chopped coriander
grated rind and juice of 1 lime

1 Mix together all the burger ingredients, except the oil. Divide the mixture into 4 and form into burgers. Cover and chill for 30 minutes.
2 Combine all the salsa ingredients in a bowl.
3 Brush the burgers with the oil and cook under a high grill or on a barbecue for about 3–4 minutes each side until cooked through.
4 Serve each burger in a bread roll with the tomato salsa and some salad leaves.

For lamb burgers, make the burgers as above but using 375 g (12 oz) lean minced lamb. Make a mint sauce by combining 5 tablespoons natural yogurt, 1 deseeded, finely chopped red chilli, 1 tablespoon roughly chopped mint and a large pinch of ground cumin.

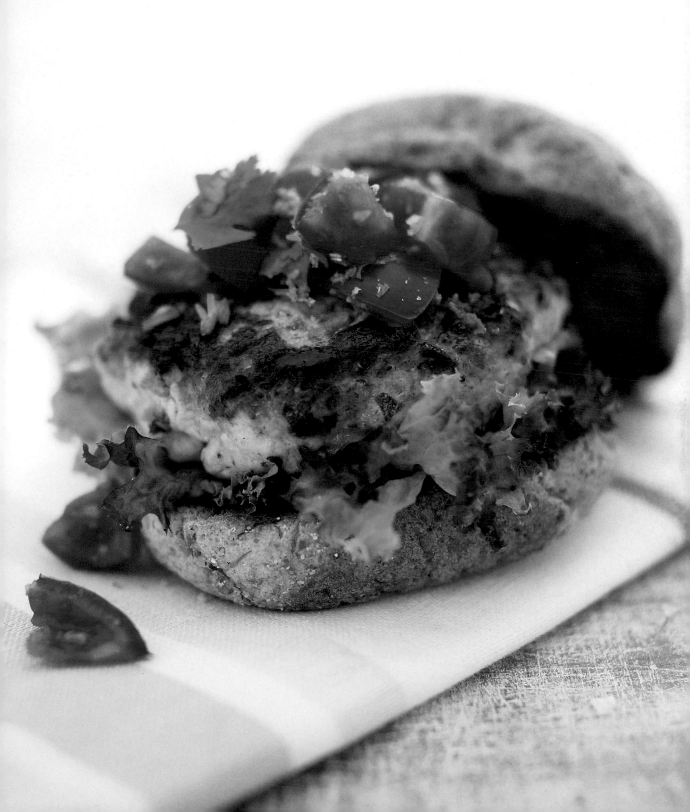

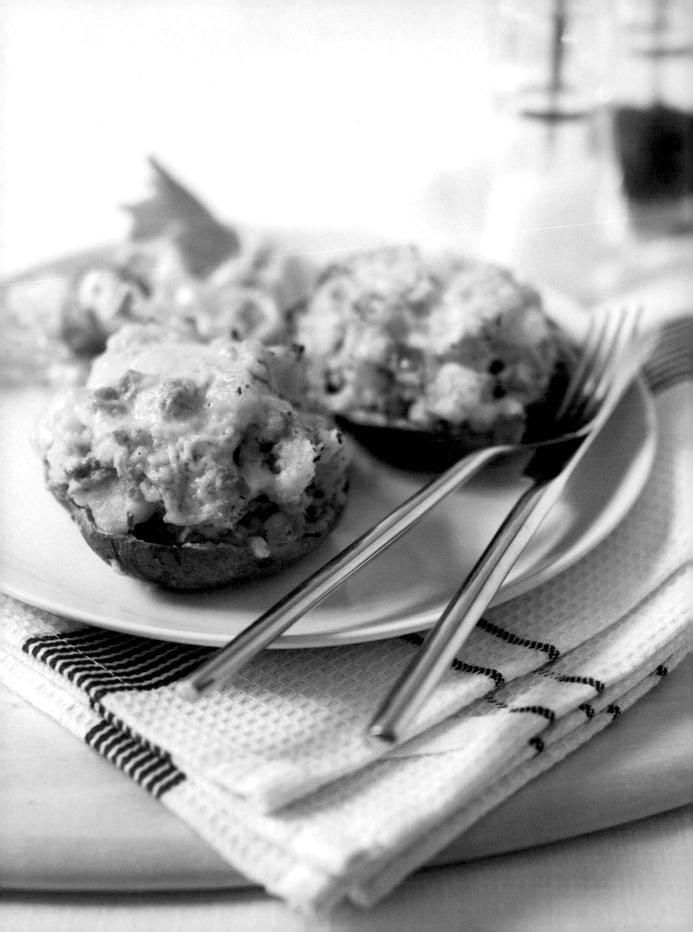

tuna & jalapeño baked potatoes

serves 4
prep + cook time 1 hour 15 minutes
+ cooling time

4 large baking potatoes
2 x 160 g (5½ oz) cans tuna in
   spring water, drained
2 tablespoons drained and
   chopped green jalapeño
   peppers in brine
2 spring onions, finely chopped
4 firm, ripe tomatoes, deseeded
   and chopped
2 tablespoons chopped chives
3 tablespoons low-fat soured
   cream
100 g (3½ oz) reduced-fat extra
   mature Cheddar cheese, grated
salt and pepper

1 Prick the potatoes all over with the tip of a sharp knife and place directly in a preheated oven, 180°C (350°F), Gas Mark 4, for 1 hour or until crisp on the outside and the inside is tender. Leave until cool enough to handle.

2 Cut the potatoes in half and scoop the cooked flesh into a bowl. Place the empty potato skins, cut side up, on a baking sheet. Mix the tuna, jalapeño peppers, spring onions, tomatoes and chives into the potato in the bowl. Gently fold in the soured cream, then season with salt and pepper to taste.

3 Spoon the filling into the potato skins, sprinkle with the Cheddar and cook under a preheated medium-hot grill for 4–5 minutes or until hot and melted. Serve immediately with a frisée salad.

Tip
Tuna packed in water is lower in fat and calories than tuna packed in oil and contains slightly higher levels of omega-3.

hummus with baked tortilla chips

serves 4
prep + cook time 17 minutes

4 small flour tortillas
1 tablespoon olive oil

hummus
400 g (13 oz) can chickpeas,
    drained and rinsed
1 garlic clove
4 tablespoons reduced-fat Greek
    yogurt
2 tablespoons lemon juice
1 tablespoon chopped coriander
    leaves
salt and pepper
paprika, to serve
coriander sprig, to garnish

1 Cut each tortilla into 8 triangles, arrange on a baking sheet and brush with a little oil. Place in a preheated oven at 200°C (400°F), Gas Mark 6 and bake for 10–12 minutes until golden and crisp. Leave to cool.

2 Meanwhile, put all the ingredients for the hummus, except the paprika and coriander, in a food processor or blender and blend until almost smooth.

3 Season to taste with salt and pepper, stir in the coriander and sprinkle with paprika. Garnish with a coriander sprig and serve with the tortilla chips.

Tip
Shop-bought tortilla chips and hummus are high in fat. This recipe is a delicious low-fat alternative.

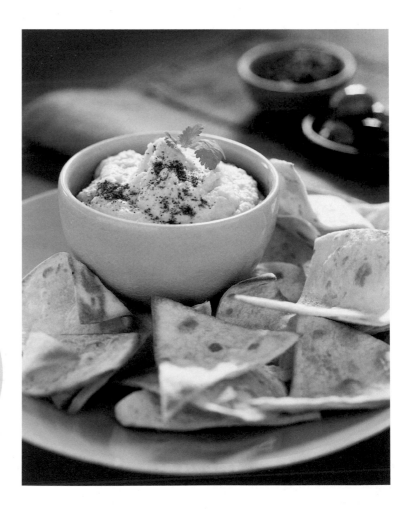

ham & poached egg toasts

serves 4
prep + cook time 20 minutes

4 thick slices of granary bread
4 slices of lean ham
2 tomatoes, sliced
4 eggs
1 tablespoon white wine vinegar
3 tablespoons reduced-fat crème
    fraîche
2 tablespoons chopped herbs,
    such as parsley or tarragon
salt and pepper

1 Toast the bread on both sides, then top each piece with a slice of ham and 2 tomato slices.
2 To poach the eggs, bring a large saucepan of water to the boil, add the vinegar, then stir the water rapidly in a circular motion to create a whirlpool. Break an egg into the centre of the pan to allow the white to wrap around the yolk. Cook for 3 minutes then remove from the pan and keep warm. Repeat with the remaining eggs, then place 1 egg on each piece of toast.
3 Mix together the crème fraîche and herbs, season to taste with salt and pepper and serve with the toasts.

Tip
Granary bread has additional wholewheat grains added to the mixture, making it rougher in texture and lower in glycaemic index.

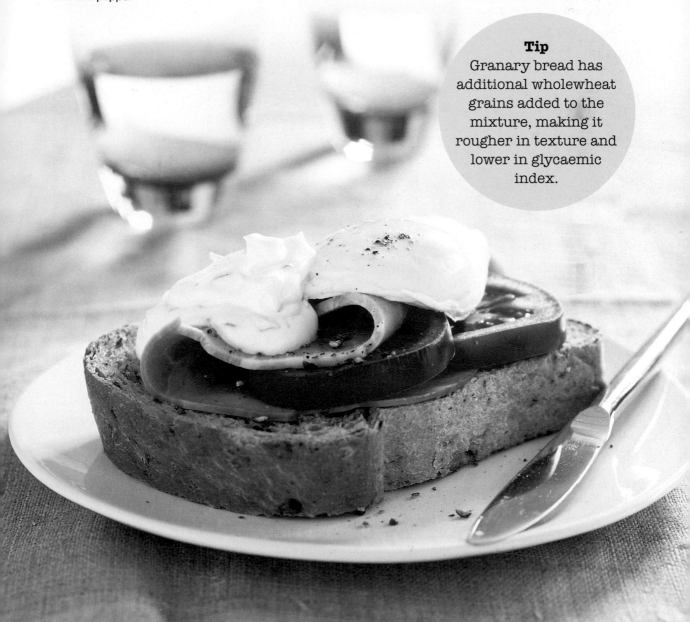

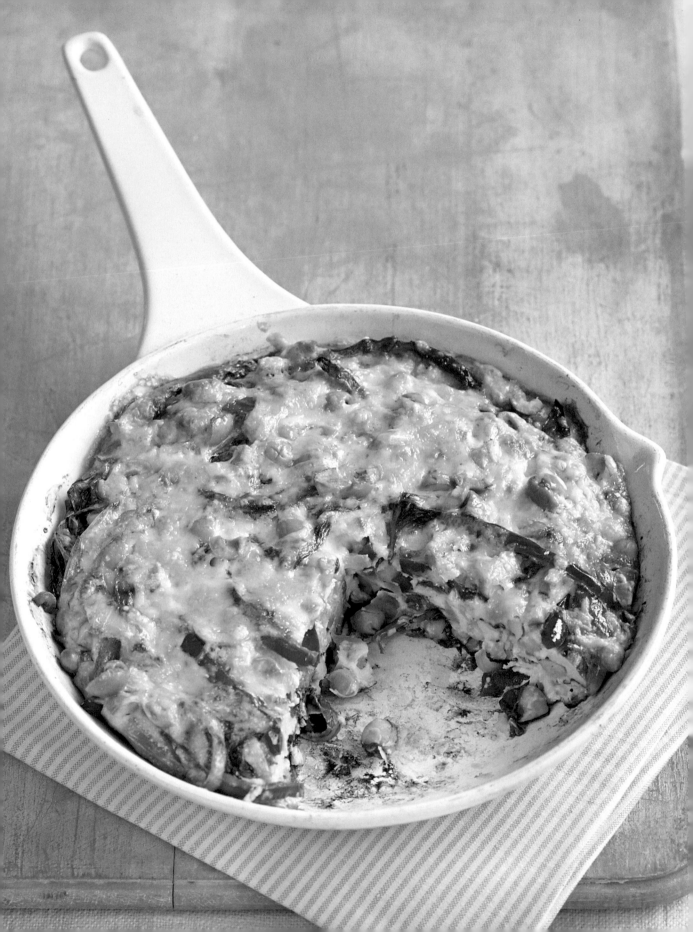

chickpea & spinach omelette

serves 4
prep + cook time 20 minutes

2 tablespoons olive oil
1 large onion, sliced
1 red pepper, sliced
½ teaspoon hot smoked or sweet
    paprika
400 g (13 oz) can chickpeas,
    drained and rinsed
100 g (3½ oz) spinach leaves,
    rinsed and roughly sliced
5 eggs, lightly beaten
75 g (3 oz) pitted green olives,
    roughly chopped
150 g (5 oz) reduced-fat Cheddar
    cheese, grated
salt and pepper

1 Heat the olive oil in a large nonstick frying pan. Add the onion and pepper and cook gently for 7–8 minutes, until soft and golden. Stir in the paprika and chickpeas, and cook for 1 minute, stirring frequently. Add the spinach leaves and cook until just wilted.

2 Pour the beaten eggs into the pan and stir to combine. Cook gently, without stirring, for 4–5 minutes, until almost set.

3 Sprinkle with the olives and grated Cheddar, then slide under a hot grill, keeping the handle away from the heat. Grill for 4–5 minutes, until golden and set. Slice into wedges and serve immediately.

Tip
Budget-friendly, eggs are full of nutrition. They are rich in vitamins B2, B12, D and A and in iodine and selenium.

smoked salmon blinis with dill cream

serves 4
prep + cook time 10 minutes

8 large blinis
2 tablespoons reduced-fat crème
   fraîche
1 teaspoon chopped dill
grated rind of 1 lemon
2 spring onions, sliced
100 g (3½ oz) smoked salmon
lemon wedges, to garnish
pepper

1 Gently warm the blinis for a few minutes under a grill or in the oven.
2 Stir together the crème fraîche, dill, lemon rind and spring onions and season with pepper. Spoon the mixture on to the blinis and top with the salmon. Garnish with lemon wedges and serve.

Tip
Reduced-fat crème fraîche is lower in fat than single cream and has a third to half of the fat of standard crème fraîche.

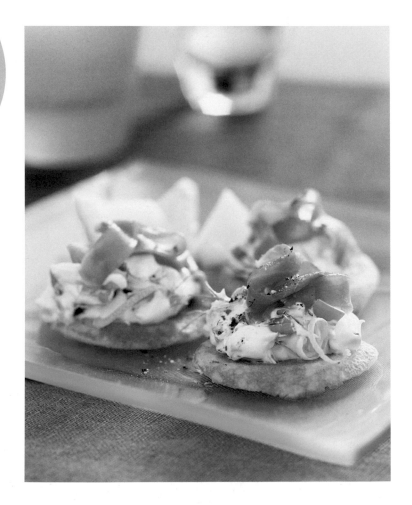

steak sandwiches

serves 4
prep + cook time 18 minutes + standing time

4 pieces thin cut sirloin steak, about 125 g (4 oz) each
1 tablespoon oil
1 onion, sliced
4 tablespoons reduced-fat crème fraîche
1 tablespoon wholegrain mustard
1 French stick, cut into 4 and split down one side
60 g (2½ oz) rocket
2 tomatoes, sliced
salt and pepper

1 Heat a griddle or nonstick frying pan until very hot.

2 Place the steak on the griddle and cook for 2 minutes on each side, or until cooked to taste. Remove the steak and leave it to rest for 5 minutes.

3 Meanwhile, add the oil to the griddle and fry the sliced onion for 2–3 minutes.

4 Mix together the crème fraîche and mustard.

5 Assemble the sandwich by placing the steak in the bread, then add the rocket, tomatoes and onion. Finish with a dollop of the mustard and crème fraîche mixture and season to taste with salt and pepper.

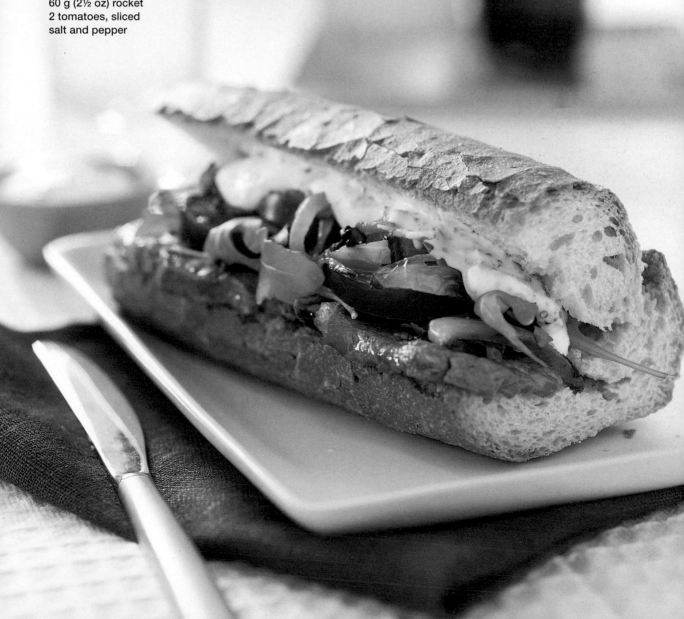

homemade baked beans

serves 4
prep + cook time 20 minutes

2 tablespoons olive or vegetable
   oil
1 onion, thinly sliced
2 garlic cloves, crushed
500 g (1 lb) passata
100 ml (3½ fl oz) hot vegetable
   stock or water
½ teaspoon sugar
2 x 400 g (13 oz) cans haricot
   beans, drained and rinsed
pinch of cayenne (optional)
pinch of cinnamon (optional)
salt and pepper
4 thick slices of granary bread,
   to serve

1 Heat the olive oil in a heavy-based saucepan and cook the onion gently for 3–4 minutes. Add the garlic and cook for a further 2 minutes, until softened and golden.

2 Add the passata, stock, sugar, beans and spices, if using, and season to taste with salt and pepper. Simmer gently for 12–14 minutes, until rich and thick.

3 Meanwhile, toast the bread until golden and place on 4 plates. Serve the beans spooned over the toast.

Tip
These super-fast homemade baked beans have very little salt and almost no sugar, making them far healthier than most shop-bought baked beans.

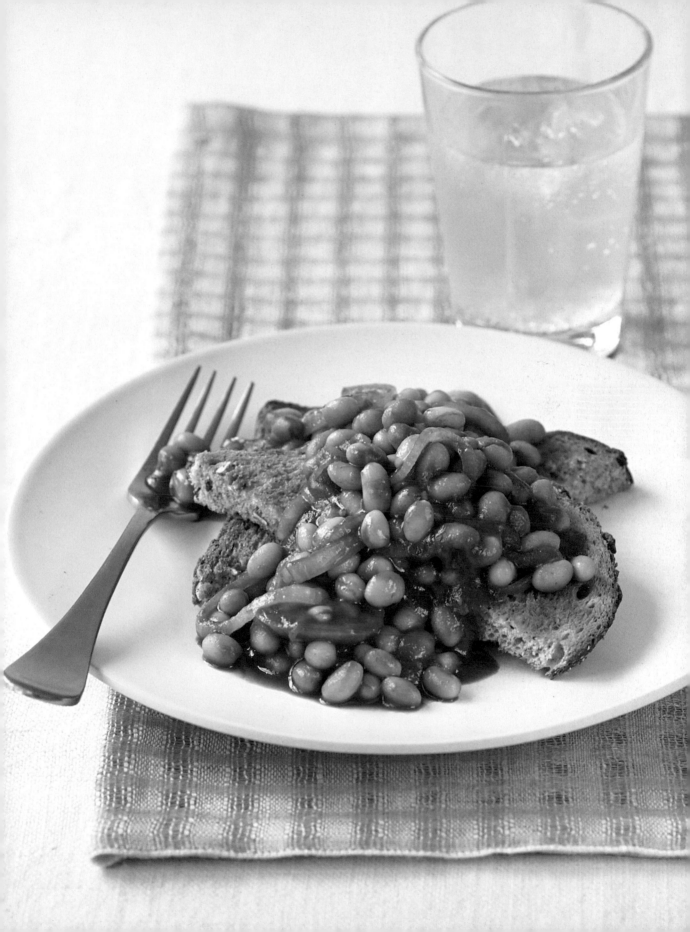

chicken fajitas

serves 4
prep + cook time 20 minutes

1 tablespoon olive oil
2 boneless, skinless chicken
   breasts, sliced
2 red onions, cut into wedges
2 red peppers, cored, deseeded
   and sliced
1 yellow pepper, cored, deseeded
   and sliced
pinch of dried chilli flakes
2 tablespoons chopped coriander
   leaves
2 tablespoons lime juice
8 medium flour tortillas
4 tablespoons reduced-fat crème
   fraîche
coriander sprigs, to garnish
60 g (2½ oz) salad leaves, to serve

1 Heat the oil in a frying pan, add the chicken and fry for 2–3 minutes until beginning to brown.
2 Add the onions, peppers and chilli flakes and continue to fry for 5 minutes more. Remove from the heat and stir in the coriander and lime juice.
3 Warm the tortillas according to the packet instructions, then fill them with the chicken mixture and crème fraîche. Garnish with coriander sprigs and serve with salad leaves.

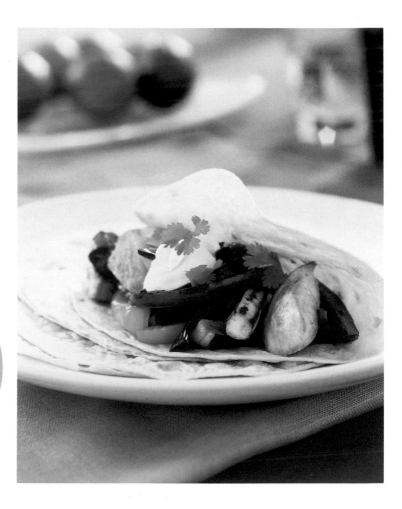

Tip
Chicken is full of vitamins and minerals and with the skin removed it is also low in fat.

lemon, mint & chicken skewers

serves 4
prep + cook time 20 minutes

150 g (5 oz) reduced-fat Greek
    yogurt
finely grated rind and juice of
    1 lemon
2 tablespoons chopped mint
2 tablespoons olive oil
4 skinless chicken breast fillets,
    each cut into 8 pieces
salt and pepper

to serve
pitta breads, warmed
cucumber, sliced
radish, sliced

1 Mix together the yogurt, lemon rind and juice, mint and olive oil. Add the chicken pieces and stir well to coat.

2 Thread the chicken on to 4 skewers and place on a foil-lined grill pan. Cook under a preheated hot grill for about 10 minutes, turning occasionally, or until the chicken is cooked and slightly charred at the edges. Slide the chicken off the skewers and serve in warm pitta breads with slices of cucumber and radish.

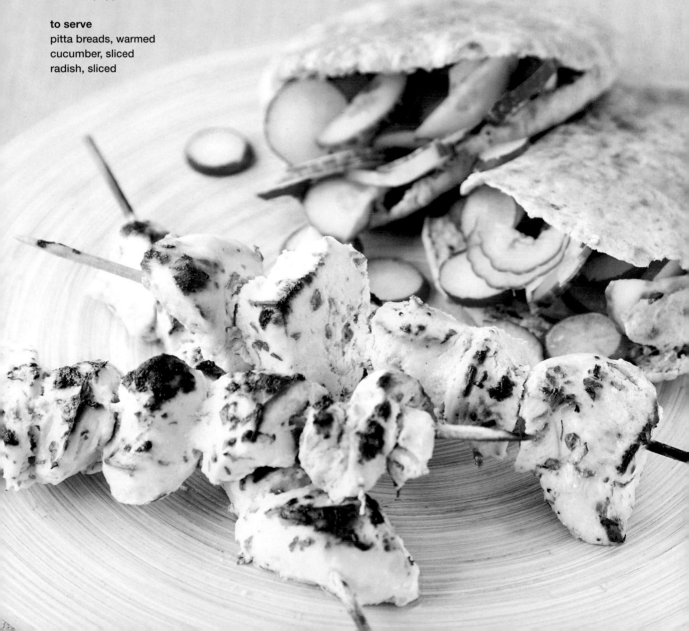

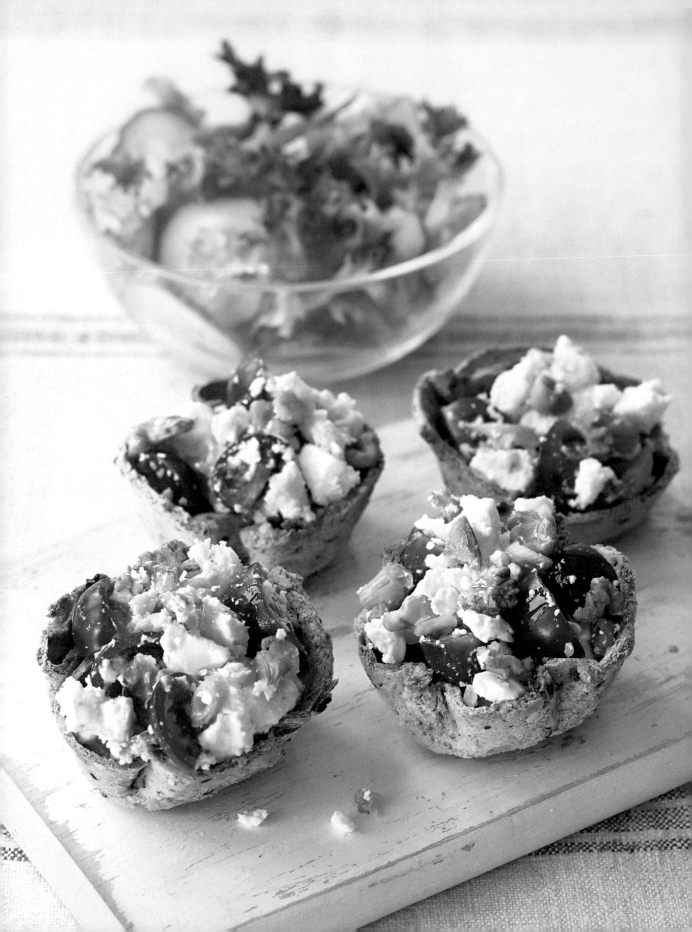

feta, spring onion & walnut tartlets

serves 4
prep + cook time 10 minutes

4 slices of brown bread, crusts
    removed
150 g (5 oz) feta cheese, crumbled
2 spring onions, thinly sliced
25 g (1 oz) walnut pieces, lightly
    crushed
8 cherry tomatoes, cut into
    quarters
1 tablespoon olive oil
salt and pepper

to serve
200 g (7 oz) mixed salad leaves
½ cucumber, sliced

1 Preheat the oven to 200°C (400°F), Gas Mark 6. Use a rolling pin to roll the bread out thinly. Cut each slice into a circle, approximately 12 cm (5 inches) in diameter, and press the circles into 4 large nonstick muffin or Yorkshire pudding tins. Cook in the preheated oven for 7–8 minutes, until crisp and golden.

2 Meanwhile, mix the crumbled feta with the spring onions, walnut pieces and tomatoes. Season to taste, then spoon the mixture into the toasted tart cases. Drizzle with the olive oil and serve with a mixed leaf and cucumber salad.

Tip
Bread tart cases are quick to make and offer a low-fat alternative to pastry. You can use a variety of fillings to make easy yet impressive party nibbles.

super smoothies

serves 4
prep time 10 minutes

strawberry
1 banana, chopped
500 g (1 lb) strawberries, hulled
900 ml (1½ pints) ice-cold
   semi-skimmed milk

peach melba
1 banana, chopped
2 peaches, stoned
250 g (8 oz) strawberries, hulled
900 ml (1½ pints) ice-cold
   semi-skimmed milk

tropical
500 g (1 lb) frozen tropical fruits,
   almost defrosted
600 ml (1 pint) ice-cold
   unsweetened pineapple juice

1 Place all the ingredients in a food processor or blender and blend until smooth.
2 Serve in tall glasses.

Tip
Smoothies are packed with vitamins and fibre and a good way of consuming the recommended daily allowance of fruit.

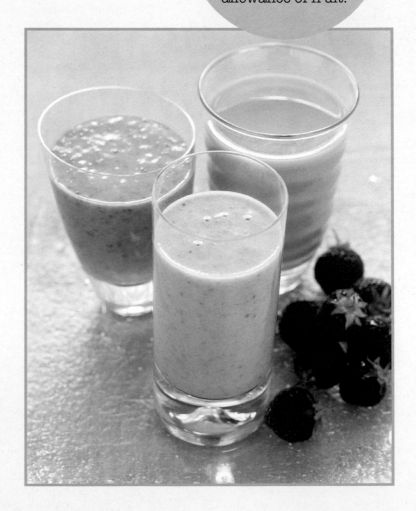

fresh figs with ricotta & parma ham

serves 4
prep time 10 minutes

8 fresh figs
1 teaspoon Dijon mustard
125 g (4 oz) ricotta cheese
85 g (3¼ oz) Parma ham, thinly
   sliced
2 tablespoons balsamic vinegar
salt and pepper
crusty bread, to serve

1 Cut the figs into 4, leaving them attached at the base.
2 Stir the mustard into the ricotta and season to taste with salt and pepper.
3 Divide the ricotta mixture between the figs, spooning it over the top. Place 2 figs on each serving plate and top with some slices of Parma ham.
4 Drizzle over the balsamic vinegar and serve the figs with crusty bread.

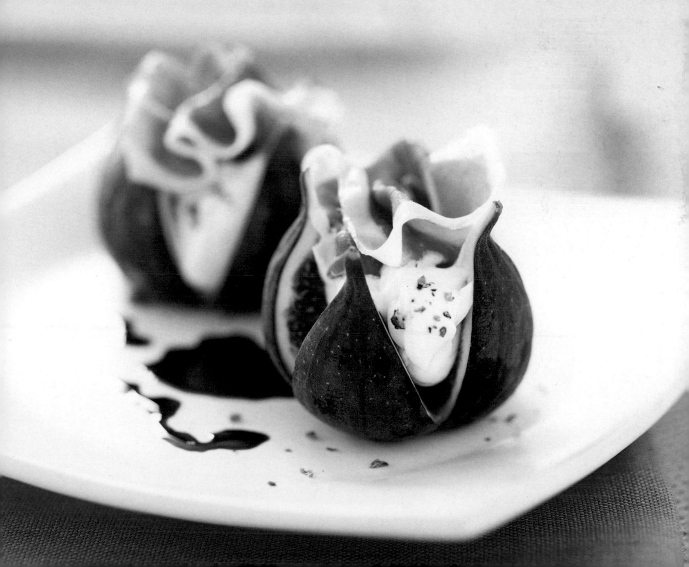

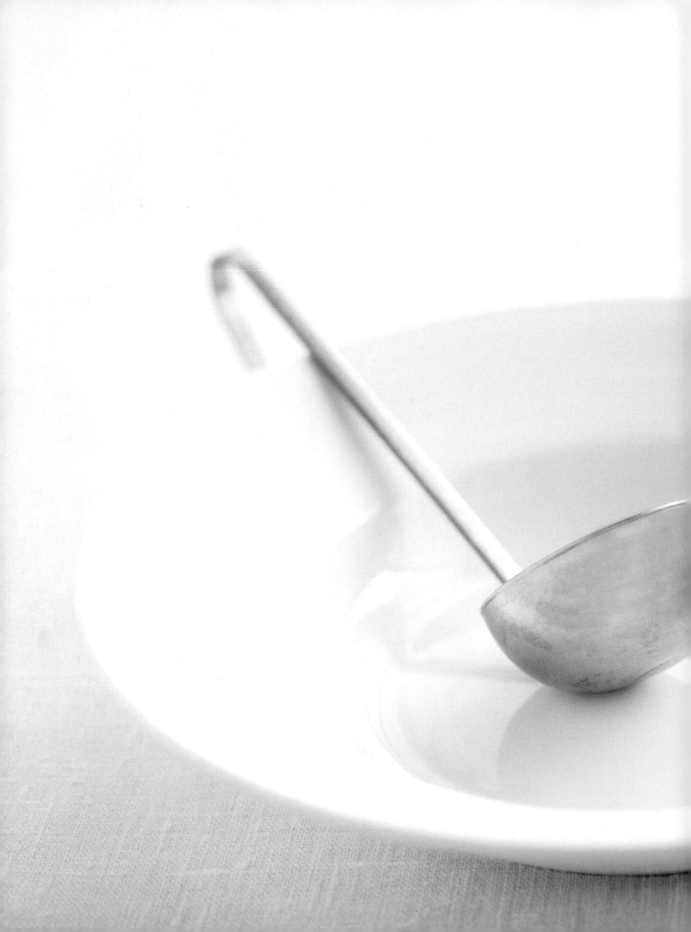

soups
& salads

smoked haddock & kale soup

serves 4
prep + cook time 30 minutes

1 tablespoon olive oil
2 shallots, diced
3 garlic cloves, crushed
1 large potato, peeled and diced
350 ml (12 fl oz) semi-skimmed
   milk
500 ml (17 fl oz) water
300 g (10 oz) kale, shredded
300 g (10 oz) smoked haddock,
   skinned and chopped
salt and pepper

1 Heat the oil in a saucepan, add the shallots and garlic and cook for 3–4 minutes until softened. Add the potato, milk and measurement water and season to taste. Bring to the boil, then reduce the heat and simmer for 5–6 minutes.
2 Stir in the kale and cook for a further 10–12 minutes until the vegetables are tender. Stir in the haddock and simmer for 2 minutes or until cooked through.
3 Ladle the soup into bowls and serve immediately.

Tip
One of the healthiest vegetables around, kale is chock-full of vitamins and minerals including vitamins B6, C and E, iron, calcium and potassium.

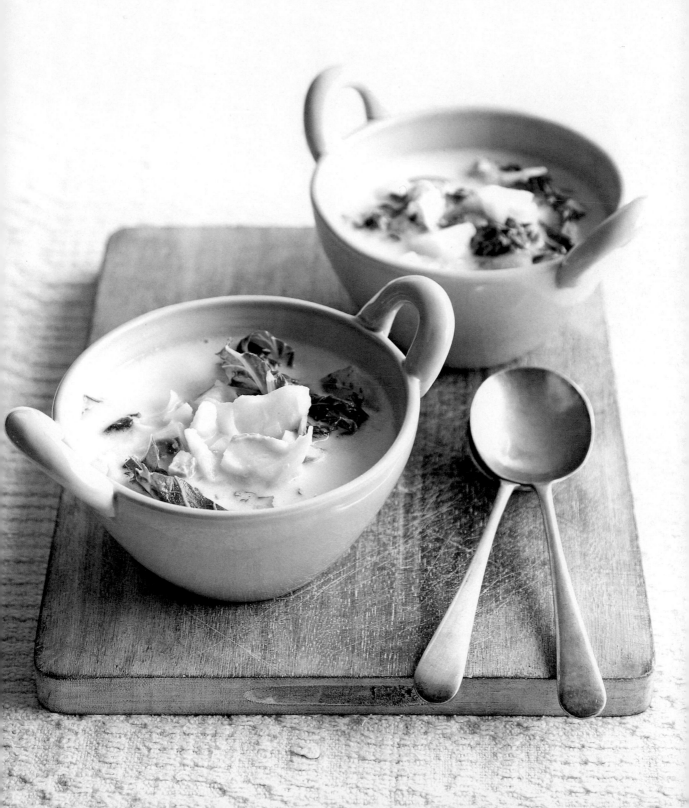

prawn & noodle soup

serves 4
prep + cook time 20 minutes

900 ml (1½ pints) vegetable or
    chicken stock
2 kaffir lime leaves
1 lemongrass stalk, lightly bruised
150 g (5 oz) dried egg noodles
50 g (2 oz) frozen peas
50 g (2 oz) frozen sweetcorn
100 g (3½ oz) large, cooked and
    peeled prawns
4 spring onions, sliced
2 teaspoons light soy sauce

1 Put the stock into a saucepan with the lime leaves and lemongrass, bring to the boil and simmer for 10 minutes.

2 Add the noodles to the stock and cook according to packet instructions. After 2 minutes, add the peas, sweetcorn, prawns, spring onions and soy sauce. Ladle into bowls and serve.

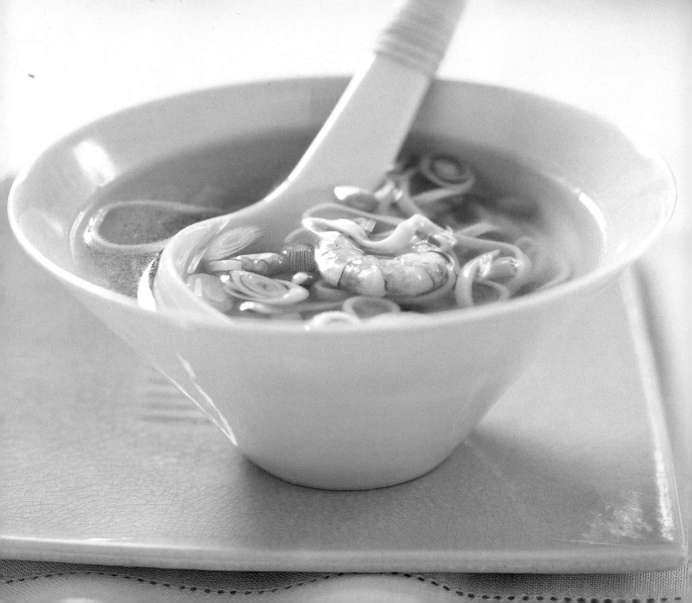

gazpacho

serves 6
prep + cook time 20 minutes + chilling time

875 g (1¾ lb) tomatoes, skinned and roughly chopped
½ cucumber, roughly chopped
2 red peppers, deseeded and roughly chopped
1 stick celery, chopped
2 garlic cloves, chopped
½ red chilli, deseeded and sliced
small handful of coriander or flat leaf parsley, plus extra to garnish
2 tablespoons white wine vinegar
2 tablespoons sun-dried tomato paste
4 tablespoons olive oil
salt

to serve
ice cubes
hard-boiled egg, finely chopped
a little cucumber, pepper and onion, finely chopped

1 Mix together the vegetables, garlic, chilli and coriander in a large bowl.

2 Add the vinegar, tomato paste, oil and a little salt. Process in batches in a food processor or blender until smooth, scraping the mixture down from the sides of the bowl if necessary.

3 Collect the blended mixtures together in a clean bowl and check the seasoning, adding a little more salt if needed. Chill for up to 24 hours before serving.

4 To serve, ladle the gazpacho into large bowls, scatter with ice cubes and garnish with chopped parsley or coriander and a little chopped hard-boiled egg, cucumber, pepper and onion, if wished.

Tip
Frozen vegetables can be just as nutritious as fresh vegetables. As well as keeping a good colour and flavour, most of the nutrients are retained.

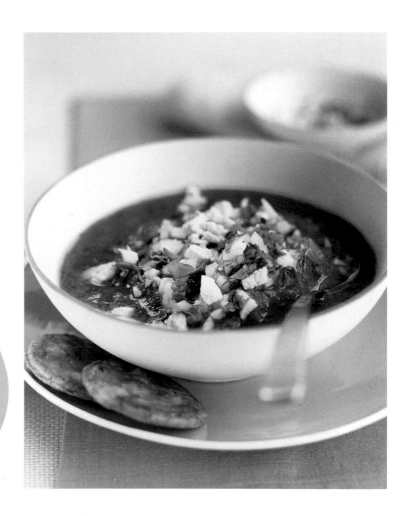

beetroot & apple soup

serves 4
prep + cook time 20 minutes

1 tablespoon olive oil
1 tablespoon butter
2 Bramley apples, peeled, cored
   and chopped
1 dessert apple, peeled, cored
   and chopped
625 g (1¼ lb) cooked beetroot,
   roughly chopped
2 teaspoons caraway seeds
4–5 fresh thyme sprigs
1.5 litres (2½ pints) vegetable
   stock
salt and pepper
reduced-fat crème fraîche, to
   serve
chopped dill, to garnish

1 Heat the oil and butter in a pan and fry the apples for 2–3 minutes until golden. Add the cooked beetroot, caraway seeds and thyme and stir-fry for 1–2 minutes.

2 Add the stock, bring to the boil then cook for 10 minutes.

3 In a blender or with a hand-held blender, whizz the soup until fairly smooth and season to taste.

4 Serve in bowls with crème fraîche swirled through. Garnish with chopped dill and freshly ground black pepper.

Tip
Blended into soups, roasted or added to salads and juices, super food beetroot is a rich source of antioxidants, minerals and vitamins.

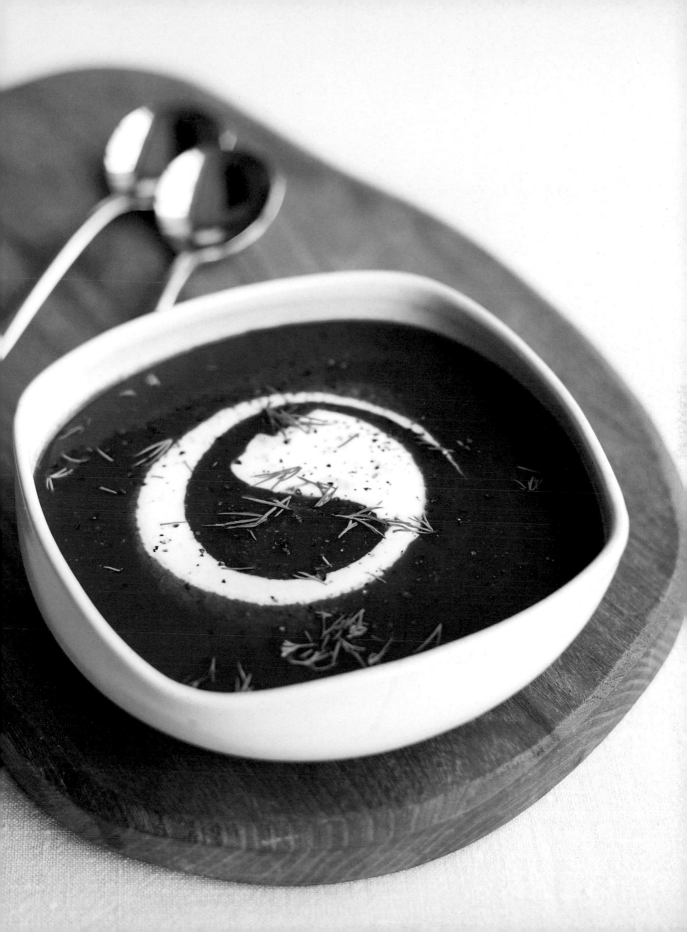

cauliflower & cumin soup

serves 4
prep + cook time 35 minutes

2 teaspoons sunflower oil
1 onion, chopped
1 garlic clove, crushed
2 teaspoons cumin seeds
1 cauliflower, cut into florets
1 large potato, peeled and
    chopped
450 ml (¾ pint) vegetable stock
450 ml (¾ pint) semi-skimmed milk
2 tablespoons reduced-fat crème
    fraîche'
2 tablespoons chopped coriander
    leaves
salt and pepper

1 Heat the oil in a medium saucepan and fry the onion, garlic and cumin seeds for 3–4 minutes. Add the cauliflower, potato, stock and milk and bring to the boil. Reduce the heat and simmer for 15 minutes.
2 Transfer the soup to a blender or food processor and purée until smooth. Stir through the crème fraîche and coriander and season to taste with salt and pepper. Heat through and serve with slices of crusty wholemeal bread.

For curried cauliflower soup, fry the onion and garlic in the oil as above, omitting the cumin. Stir in 2 tablespoons mild curry paste, cook for 1 minute then add the cauliflower, potato, stock and milk. Continue as the recipe above.

summer green pea soup

serves 4
prep + cook time 25 minutes (or longer if shelling fresh peas)

1 tablespoon butter
bunch of spring onions, chopped
1.25 kg (2½ lb) fresh peas, shelled, or 500 g (1 lb) frozen peas
750 ml (1¼ pints) vegetable stock
2 tablespoons reduced-fat natural yogurt
nutmeg
1 tablespoon chopped and 2 whole chives, to garnish

1 Melt the butter in a large pan and soften the onions, but do not allow them to colour. Add the peas to the pan with the stock. Bring to the boil and simmer for about 5 minutes for frozen peas, but for up to 15 minutes for fresh peas, until they are cooked. Be careful not to overcook fresh peas or they will lose their flavour.

2 Remove from the heat and purée in a blender or food processor. Add the yogurt and grate in a little nutmeg. Reheat gently if necessary, and serve sprinkled with chives.

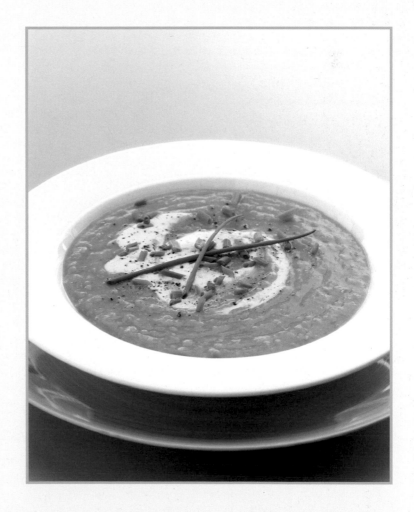

spicy coriander & lentil soup

serves 8
prep + cook time 1 hour to 1 hour 15 minutes

500 g (1 lb) red lentils
2 tablespoons vegetable oil
2 onions, chopped
2 garlic cloves, chopped
2 celery sticks, chopped
400 g (13 oz) can tomatoes, drained
1 chilli, deseeded and chopped (optional)
1 teaspoon paprika
1 teaspoon harissa paste
1 teaspoon ground cumin
1.2 litres (2 pints) vegetable stock
salt and pepper
2 tablespoons chopped coriander, to garnish

1 Place the lentils in a bowl of water. Heat the oil in a large saucepan and gently fry the onions, garlic and celery over a low heat until softened.

2 Drain the lentils and add them to the vegetable pan with the tomatoes. Mix well. Add the chilli, if using, paprika, harissa paste, cumin and vegetable stock and season with salt and pepper. Cover the pan and simmer gently for about 40–50 minutes until the lentils are tender, adding a little more vegetable stock or water if the soup gets too thick.

3 Serve the soup immediately topped with a little chopped coriander.

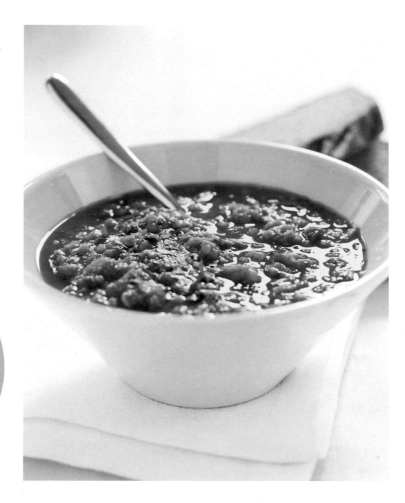

Tip
A great way to add fibre, protein and iron to your diet, versatile lentils can be used in soups, stews, curries and salads.

miso chicken broth

serves 4
prep + cook time 30 minutes

1 tablespoon sunflower oil
2 boneless, skinless chicken
   breasts, diced
250 g (8 oz) cup mushrooms,
   sliced
1 carrot, cut into thin matchsticks
1.5 cm (¾ inch) piece root ginger,
   grated
2 large pinches dried crushed red
   chillies
2 tablespoons brown rice miso
   paste
4 tablespoons mirin or dry sherry
2 tablespoons light soy sauce
1.2 litres (2 pints) water
2 pak choi, thinly sliced
4 spring onions, thinly sliced
4 tablespoons fresh chopped
   coriander

1 Heat the oil in a saucepan, add the chicken and fry for 4–5 minutes, stirring until golden. Add the mushrooms and carrot sticks, then the ginger, chillies, miso, mirin or sherry and soy sauce.
2 Pour on the water and bring to the boil, stirring. Simmer for 10 minutes.
3 Add the pak choi, spring onions and chopped coriander and cook for 2–3 minutes until the pak choi has just wilted. Spoon into bowls and serve.

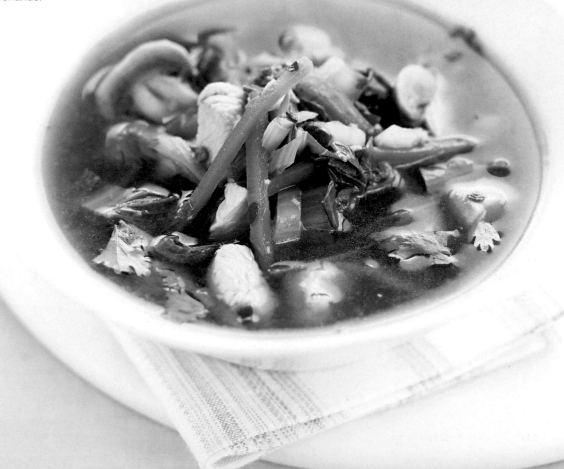

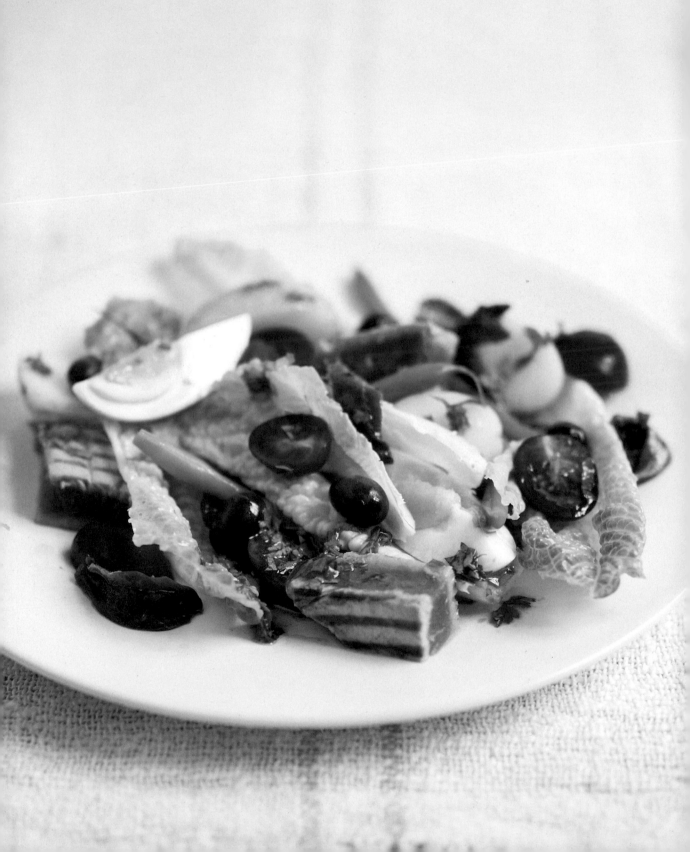

seared tuna with niçoise salad

serves 4
prep + cook time 30 minutes

300 g (10 oz) salad potatoes,
    halved
2 eggs
100 g (3½ oz) green beans
1 tablespoon olive oil
450 g (14½ oz) piece of very
    fresh tuna
125 g (4 oz) cherry tomatoes,
    halved
2 cos lettuces
8 anchovy fillets in oil, drained
75 g (3 oz) black olives
salt and pepper

vinaigrette
2 garlic cloves, crushed
1 teaspoon Dijon mustard
1 tablespoon red wine vinegar
1 tablespoon lemon juice
6 tablespoons extra virgin olive oil
handful of parsley, chopped

1 Cook the potatoes in a saucepan of lightly salted boiling water for 12–15 minutes until just tender. Drain and cool under cold running water. Meanwhile, gently lower the eggs into a saucepan of boiling water and cook for 8 minutes. Drain and cool as before, then shell. Cook the beans in a saucepan of lightly salted boiling water for 5 minutes until just tender. Drain and cool as before.

2 Meanwhile, mix together all the ingredients for the vinaigrette and season well. Toss half the vinaigrette with the potatoes and beans and set aside. Rub the oil over the tuna and season well. Heat a griddle pan until smoking hot and cook for 2 minutes on each side until browned but still rare inside. Cut into bite-sized pieces.

3 Toss the tomatoes with the potatoes and beans. Separate the leaves of the lettuces, then arrange on a serving plate with the anchovies, olives, eggs, quartered, the tuna slices and drizzle over the remaining dressing.

Tip
Idea for char-grilling, fresh tuna is an excellent source of protein and omega-3 fatty acids.

spring vegetable salad

serves 4
prep + cook time 20 minutes

200 g (7 oz) fresh or frozen peas
200 g (7 oz) asparagus, trimmed
200 g (7 oz) sugar snap peas
2 courgettes
1 fennel bulb

dressing
grated rind and juice of 1 lemon
1 teaspoon Dijon mustard
1 teaspoon clear honey
1 tablespoon chopped flat leaf
    parsley
1 tablespoon olive oil

1 Put the peas, asparagus and sugar snap peas in a saucepan of lightly salted boiling water and simmer for 3 minutes. Drain, then refresh under cold running water.
2 Cut the courgettes into long, thin ribbons and thinly slice the fennel. Transfer all the vegetables to a large salad bowl and mix together.
3 Make the dressing by whisking together the lemon rind and juice, mustard, honey, parsley and oil in another bowl. Toss the dressing through the vegetables and serve.

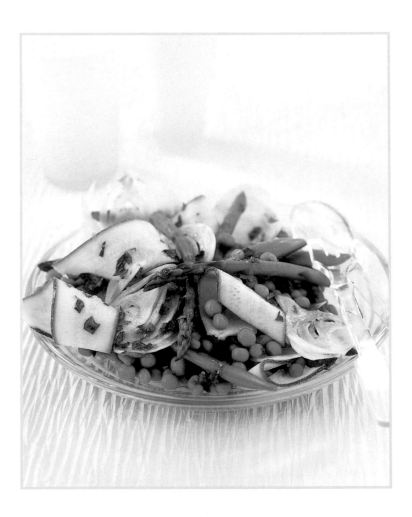

summer vegetable salad

serves 4
prep + cook time 10 minutes + marinating time

2 courgettes
2 carrots
150 g (5 oz) mangetout, halved
   lengthways
1 red pepper, cored, deseeded
   and sliced
150 g (5 oz) bean sprouts
1 red chilli, finely sliced
4 tablespoons chopped coriander
   leaves
2 tablespoons sesame seeds,
   toasted
1 tablespoon sesame oil
grated rind and juice of 1 lime

1 Use a vegetable peeler to slice the courgettes and the carrots into fine ribbons. Place them in a pan of boiling water, then immediately drain and refresh under cold running water.
2 Toss the courgette and carrot ribbons with the mangetout, red pepper, bean sprouts, chilli, coriander, sesame seeds, oil and lime rind and juice. Set aside for 20 minutes to allow the flavours to infuse. Serve in a large bowl.

Tip
Chillies owe their heat to the phytochemical capsaicin, which is concentrated in the seeds and can help relieve nasal congestion. They are also rich in vitamin C.

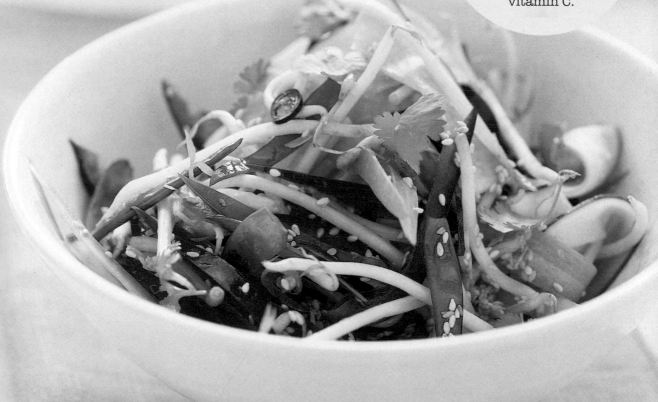

raspberry salad with toasties

serves 4
prep + cook time 20 minutes

½ red onion, thinly sliced
125 g (4 oz) mixed salad leaves,
   including baby red chard leaves
100 g (3½ oz) fresh raspberries
2 tablespoons balsamic vinegar
1 pomegranate
8 slices, about 75 g (3 oz),
   wholemeal French bread
250 g (8 oz) cottage cheese
little paprika

1 Put the onion in a bowl with the salad leaves and raspberries. Drizzle over the vinegar and toss together.
2 Cut the pomegranate into quarters, flex the skin and pop out the seeds. Sprinkle half the seeds over the salad, then transfer the salad to 4 serving plates.
3 Toast the bread on both sides and arrange 2 slices in the centre of each serving plate. Spoon the cottage cheese on to the toast, sprinkle with the remaining pomegranate seeds and a little paprika and serve.

For raspberry salad dressing, blend together 100 g raspberries, 100 ml raspberry vinegar, 150 ml olive oil, 1 teaspoon each caster sugar and Dijon mustard, 2 tablespoons chopped tarragon and 1 chopped garlic clove. Season to taste.

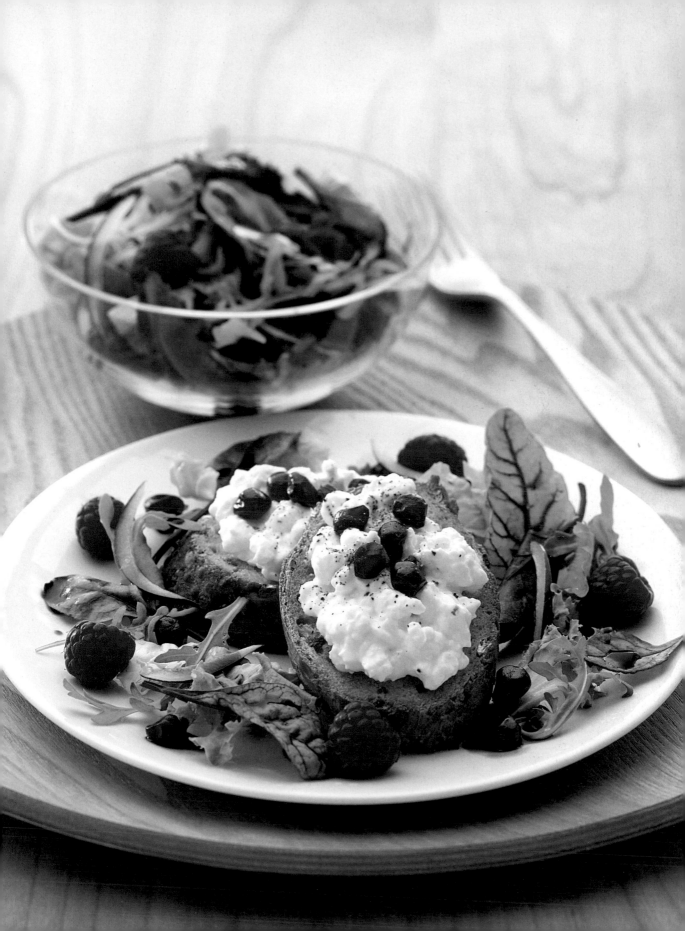

warm aubergine salad

serves 4
prep + cook time 20 minutes + cooling time

2 tablespoons olive oil
2 aubergines, cut into small cubes
1 red onion, finely sliced
2 tablespoons capers, roughly chopped
4 tomatoes, chopped
4 tablespoons chopped parsley
1 tablespoon balsamic vinegar

to serve
salad leaves
fresh crusty bread

1 Heat the oil in a nonstick frying pan. Add the aubergines and fry for 10 minutes until golden and softened. Add the red onion, capers, tomatoes, parsley and vinegar and stir to combine.
2 Remove the pan from the heat and leave to cool for 10 minutes. Serve the aubergine salad with salad leaves and crusty bread.

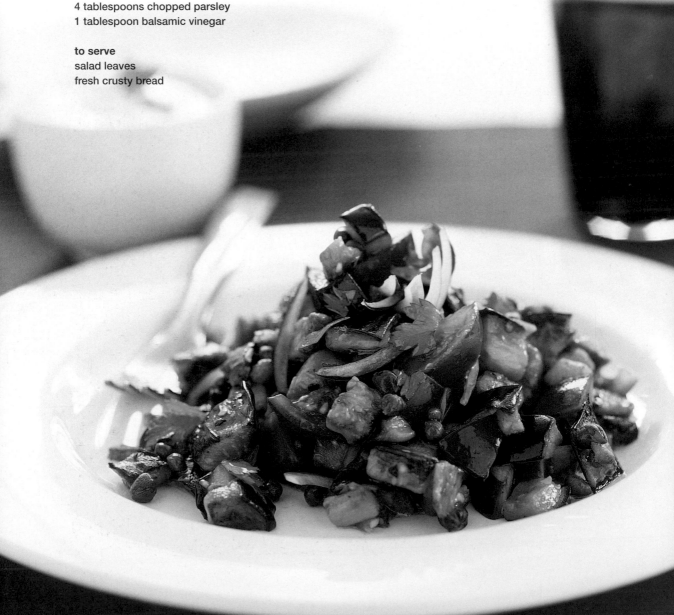

pearl barley salad with griddled chicken

serves 4
prep + cook time 20 minutes

4 boneless, skinless chicken
    breasts
1 tablespoon olive oil
125 g (4 oz) pearl barley, cooked
    according to packet instructions
1 red onion, finely chopped
1 red chilli, finely chopped
4 tablespoons chopped coriander
    leaves
grated rind and juice of 2 limes
1 red pepper, cored, deseeded
    and finely chopped
salt and pepper
parsley sprigs and lime wedges,
    to garnish

1 Brush each chicken piece with a little oil. Heat a griddle until hot and cook the chicken for 4–5 minutes on each side until cooked and browned. Cut each breast into 4 slices.

2 Stir the remaining oil into the barley, and add the onion, chilli, coriander, lime rind and juice, and red pepper. Season to taste with salt and pepper and stir to combine.

3 Serve the barley topped with the chicken, garnished with parsley and lime wedges.

Tip
Pearl barley is high in soluble fibre and can be used as a substitute for rice.

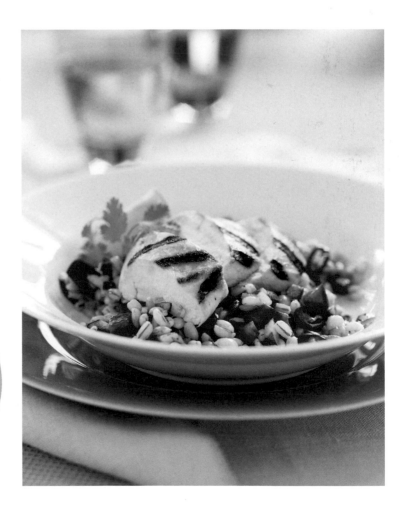

thai beef & noodle salad

serves 4
prep + cook time 30 minutes

250 g (8 oz) piece lean sirloin steak
150 g (5 oz) bean sprouts
1 red pepper, cored, deseeded and
   finely sliced
½ cucumber, peeled, deseeded
   and sliced
60 g (2½ oz) rocket
200 g (7 oz) dried egg noodles,
   cooked according to packet
   instructions

dressing
grated rind and juice of 1 lime
1 tablespoon sesame oil
1 tablespoon Thai fish sauce
1 red chilli, deseeded and finely
   sliced
4 tablespoons chopped coriander
   leaves

1 Heat a griddle or frying pan until very hot. Add the steak and fry for 1–2 minutes on each side, depending how you prefer your meat cooked. Remove from the heat and leave to rest for about 5 minutes.
2 Toss the bean sprouts, red pepper, cucumber and rocket with the noodles.
3 Mix together the dressing ingredients, pour over the salad and combine well. Divide between 4 plates.
4 Slice the steak into thin strips and place on top of the individual salads, then serve.

Tip
Lean red meat is low in fat and calories; it is also a good source of iron.

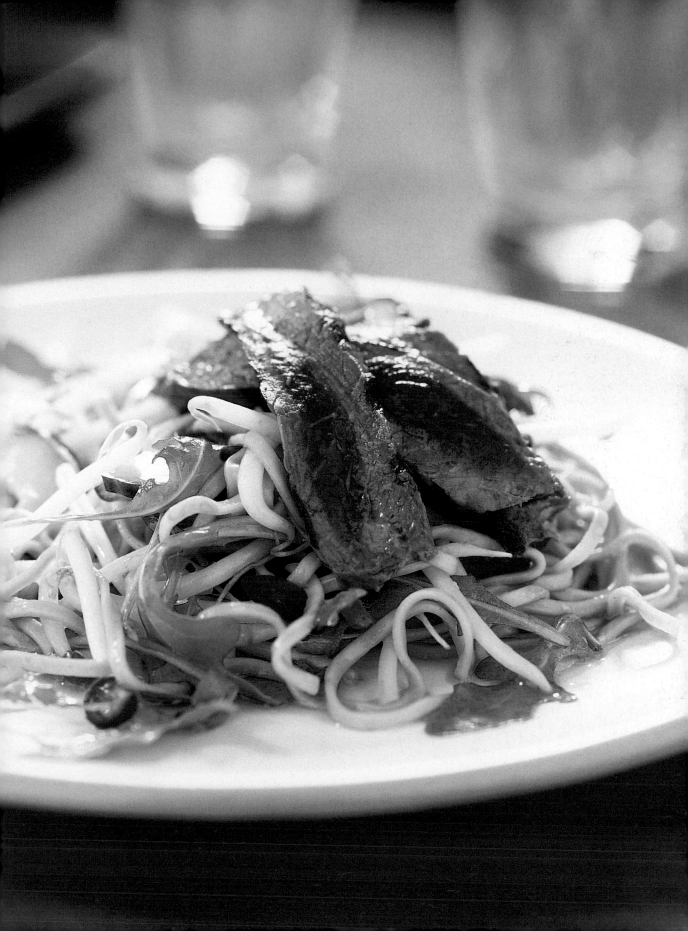

moroccan tomato & chickpea salad

serves 4
prep time 10 minutes + standing time

1 red onion, finely sliced
2 x 400 g (13 oz) cans chickpeas, drained and rinsed
4 tomatoes, chopped
4 tablespoons lemon juice
1 tablespoon olive oil
handful of herbs, such as mint and parsley, chopped
pinch of paprika
pinch of ground cumin
salt and pepper

1 Mix together all the ingredients in a large non-metallic bowl. Set aside for 10 minutes to allow the flavours to infuse, then serve.

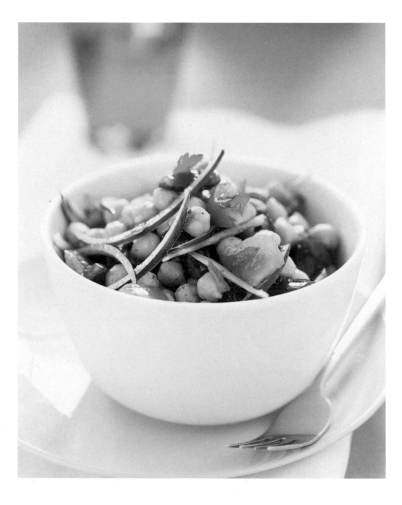

Tip
Red onions are a good source of flavonols which act as antioxidants.

mini falafel salad

serves 4
prep + cook time 20 minutes

2 x 400 g (13 oz) cans chickpeas,
   drained and rinsed
2 teaspoons ground coriander
2 teaspoons ground cumin
2 garlic cloves, crushed
2 tablespoons chopped coriander
   leaves
1 egg yolk, beaten
2 tablespoons oil
toasted mini pitta breads, to serve

salad
3 little gem lettuces, torn into
   bite-sized pieces
½ cucumber, sliced

dressing
300 g (10 oz) reduced-fat natural
   yogurt
3 tablespoons chopped mint
3 tablespoons chopped parsley
salt and pepper

1 Place two-thirds of the chickpeas in a food processor or blender with the ground coriander, cumin and garlic and blend until almost smooth. Stir in the coriander leaves and the egg yolk.
2 Form the mixture into 16 small balls and brush with the oil. Place under a preheated hot grill and grill for 3–4 minutes until golden.
3 Divide the lettuce, cucumber, the remaining chickpeas and the falafel between 4 plates.
4 Mix together the dressing ingredients. Serve the falafel salad with the dressing and the pitta breads.

Tip
Falafel are generally fried in oil; these mini falafel are lower in fat as they are brushed with oil and baked. Serve with the yogurt dressing, which is low in fat, high in protein and rich in vitamins.

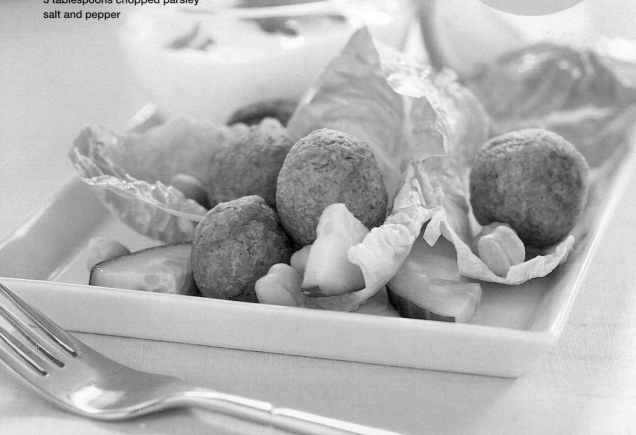

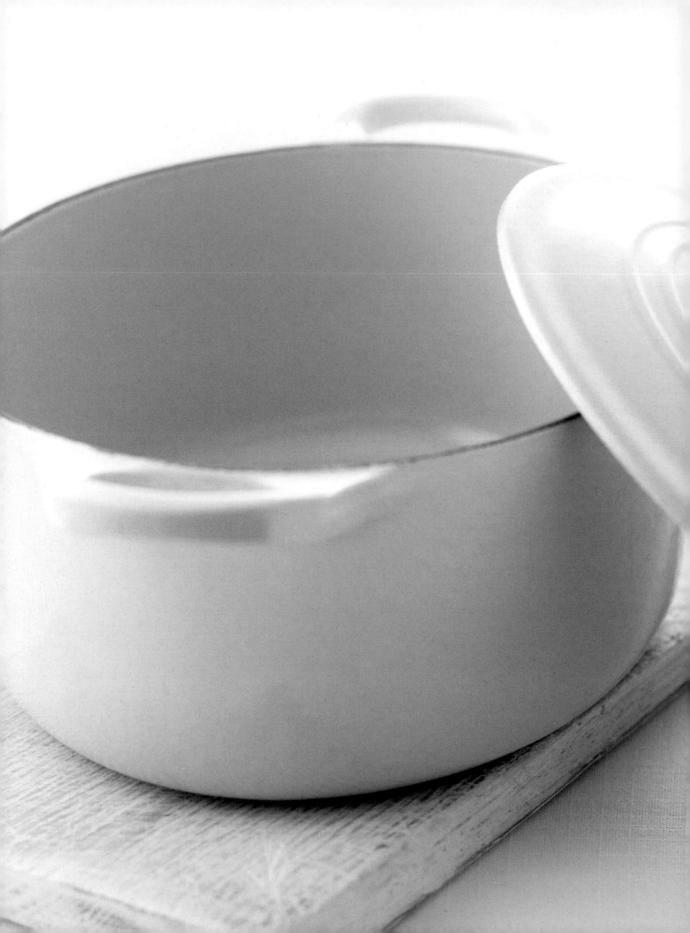

midweek favourites

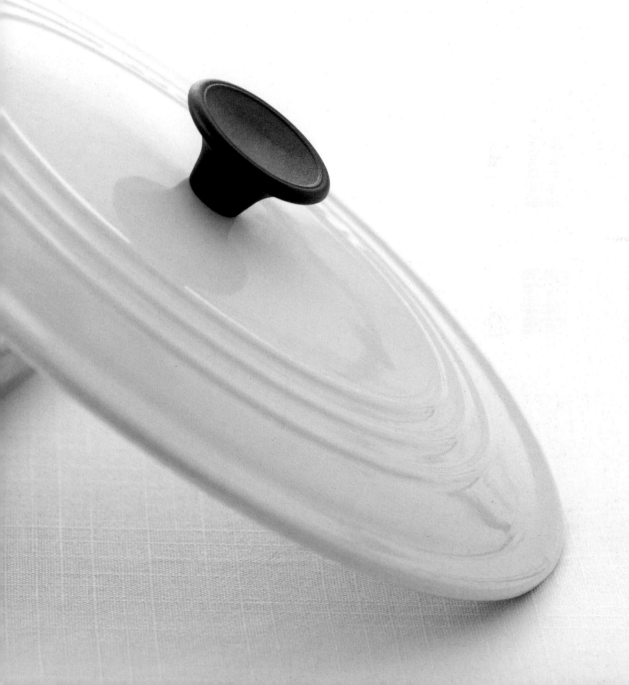

chicken & winter vegetable tray-roast

serves 4
prep + cook time 30 minutes

4 tablespoons olive oil
4 chicken breasts, skin on
400 g (13 oz) small waxy potatoes, halved
400 g (13 oz) carrots, quartered
400 g (13 oz) parsnips, cored and quartered
4 banana shallots, quartered
6 small garlic cloves
2 thyme sprigs
rosemary sprig
salt and pepper
steamed kale, to serve (optional)

1 Heat half the oil in a large frying pan over a medium-high heat and cook the chicken, skin-side down without moving, for 7–8 minutes, until the skin is really crisp and golden.

2 Meanwhile, parboil the potatoes in a large pan of lightly salted boiling water for 6–7 minutes, adding the carrots and parsnips for the final 3 minutes. They should all be starting to soften.

3 Drain well and place in a large roasting tin. Add the shallots, garlic, herbs and remaining oil, season generously and toss well. Nestle the chicken in with the vegetables, skin-side up.

4 Roast in a preheated oven, 220°C (425°F), Gas Mark 7, for about 20 minutes, until the chicken is cooked and the vegetables are golden. Serve with steamed kale, if desired.

Tip
This comforting dish is a perfect family winter warmer. Blitz any leftover roasted vegetables with vegetable stock to make a quick and easy soup.

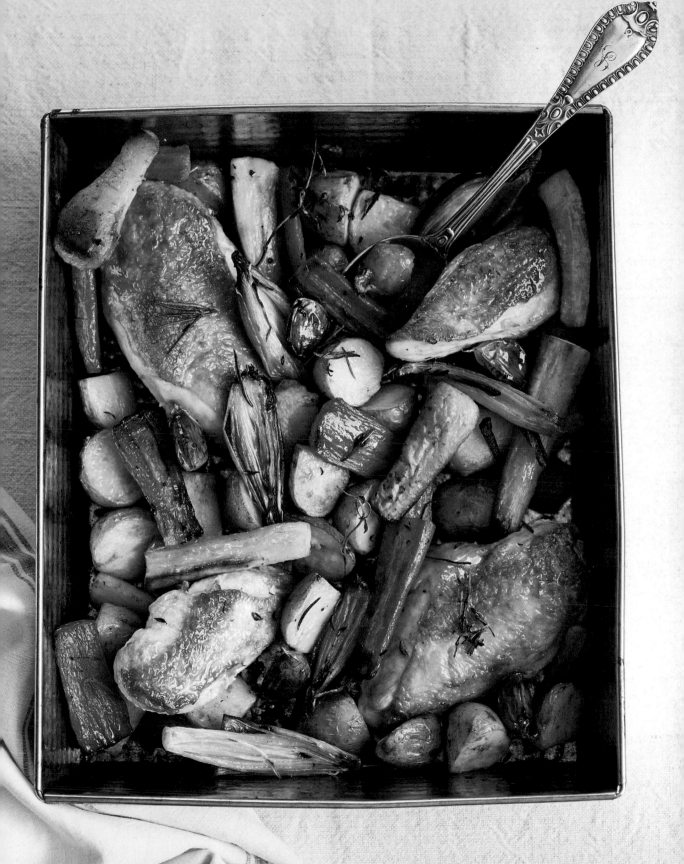

chicken drumstick jambalaya

serves 4
prep + cook time 30 minutes

1 tablespoon sunflower oil
8 chicken drumsticks, skinned
1 onion, chopped
2 garlic cloves, crushed
2 celery sticks, sliced
1 red chilli, deseeded and
    chopped
1 green pepper, cored, deseeded
    and chopped
75 g (3 oz) chorizo sausage, sliced
250 ml (8 fl oz) American long grain
    rice
500 ml (17 fl oz) chicken stock
1 bay leaf
3 tomatoes, cut into wedges
dash of Tabasco sauce
salt and pepper

1 Heat the oil in a large pan. Cut a few slashes across the thickest part of the drumsticks, add them to the pan and fry over a high heat for 5 minutes, turning occasionally. Add the onion, garlic, celery, chilli and pepper and cook for a further 2–3 minutes or until softened.
2 Add the chorizo, fry briefly, then add the rice, stirring to coat the grains in the pan juices. Pour in the stock, add the bay leaf and bring to the boil. Cover, reduce the heat and simmer for 20 minutes, stirring occasionally, until the stock has been absorbed and the rice is tender.
3 Stir in the tomatoes and Tabasco sauce and season to taste. Heat through for 3 minutes before serving.

Tip
This Cajun-inspired dish is super fast and super easy. Add a dash or two more of the Tabasco sauce if you like things extra spicy.

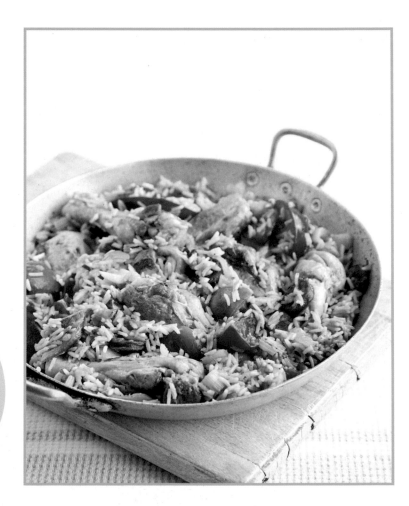

pan-fried lamb with spiced haricot beans

serves 4
prep + cook time 22 minutes
+ marinating time

½ teaspoon ground cumin
½ teaspoon ground coriander
pinch of chilli powder
1 tablespoon oil
4 lean lamb steaks
1 onion, sliced
1 garlic clove, crushed
4 tablespoons lemon juice
400 g (13 oz) can haricot beans,
    drained and rinsed
1 tablespoon chopped mint
2 tablespoons reduced-fat crème
    fraîche
salad leaves or fresh vegetables,
    to serve

1 Mix together the cumin, coriander, chilli and half the oil in a non-metallic bowl. Add the lamb, coat it in the spices and set aside for 10 minutes.
2 Heat the remaining oil in a nonstick pan, add the onion and garlic and fry for 3–4 minutes until softened.
3 Add the lamb and the marinade and fry for 2–3 minutes on each side, or until cooked to your liking.
4 Add the lemon juice, haricot beans, mint and crème fraîche and simmer for 1 minute until warmed through. Serve with salad leaves or fresh vegetables.

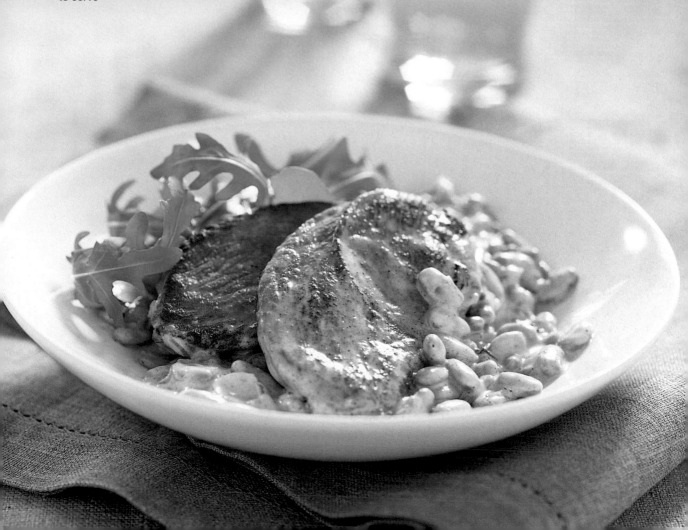

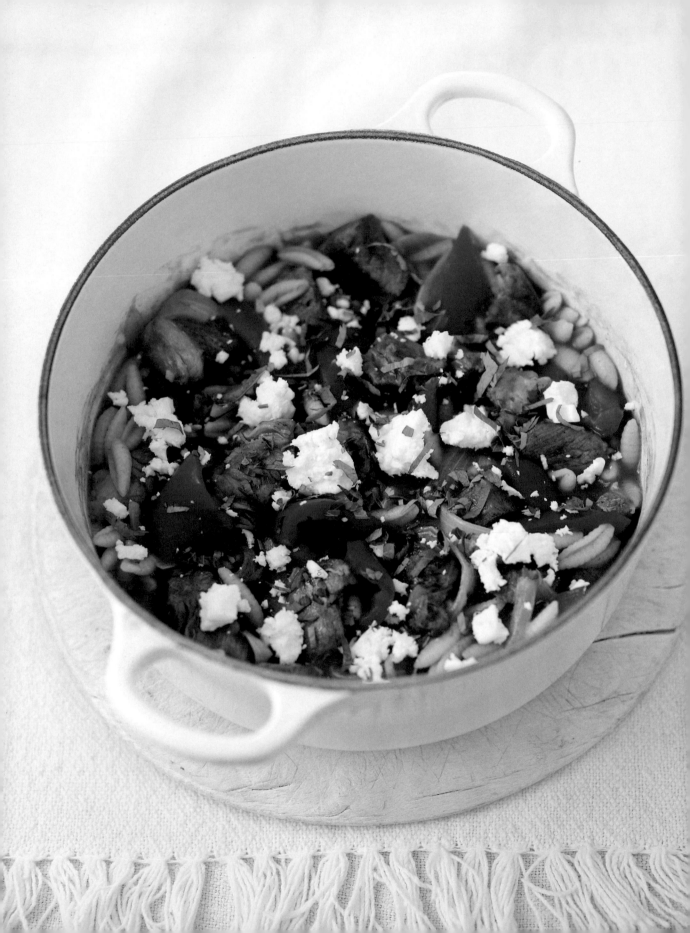

lamb stew with feta & pasta

serves 4
prep + cook time 30 minutes

2 tablespoons olive oil
400 g (13 oz) lamb fillet or neck,
    cut into bite-sized pieces
1 onion, sliced
2 garlic cloves, crushed
1 tablespoon tomato purée
½ teaspoon ground cinnamon
pinch of dried chilli flakes
1 red pepper, cored, deseeded and
    sliced
750 ml (1¼ pints) hot chicken
    stock
300 g (10 oz) small soup pasta
salt and pepper
25 g (1 oz) feta cheese, crumbled
handful of chopped parsley,
    to garnish

1 Heat the oil in a large flameproof casserole dish. Add the lamb and cook for 5 minutes until starting to brown, then add the onion and cook for a further 7–8 minutes until soft. Stir in the garlic, tomato purée, spices and red pepper, then pour in the stock.
2 Bring to the boil, then reduce the heat and simmer for 1–2 minutes, then add the pasta and cook for 12 minutes, or according to the pack instructions, until the pasta is tender and most of the liquid has boiled away. Season to taste, then serve sprinkled with the feta and parsley.

tenderloin of pork with pear & potato

serves 4
prep + cook time 35 minutes

500 g (1 lb) piece pork tenderloin
2 garlic cloves, cut into slivers
1 tablespoon seasoned flour
1 tablespoon oil
150 ml (¼ pint) dry cider
500 g (1 lb) new potatoes,
    parboiled
2 pears, quartered and cored
2 thyme sprigs
3 tablespoons reduced-fat crème
    fraîche
salt and pepper
steamed vegetables or salad,
    to serve

1 Make a few small cuts in the tenderloin with a sharp knife and push a sliver of garlic into each cut. Rub the pork all over with the seasoned flour.

2 Heat the oil in a frying pan, add the pork and fry for 3–4 minutes over a moderate heat until browned on all sides. Add the cider and simmer until reduced by half.

3 Transfer the pork and juices to a shallow ovenproof dish with the potatoes, pears and thyme.

4 Bake the dish in a preheated oven at 200°C (400°F), Gas Mark 6 for 20 minutes or until the pork is cooked through and the potatoes are tender. Stir the crème fraîche through the cooking juices and season to taste with salt and pepper. Serve with steamed vegetables or a salad.

Tip
Choose a lean piece of pork which is low in fat and remove any visible fat before cooking.

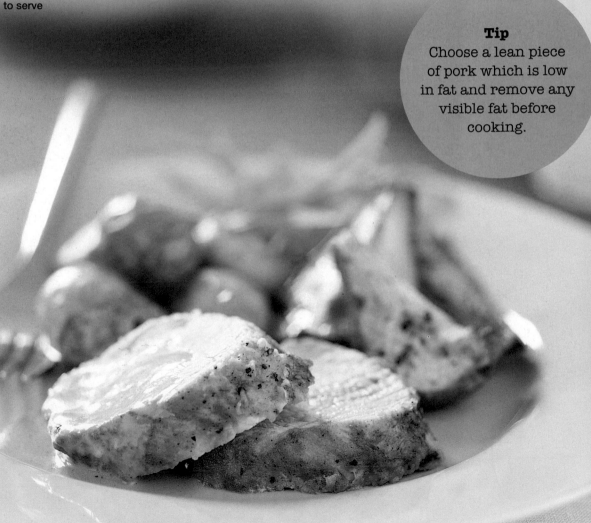

pan-fried calves' liver with mustard & sage mash

serves 4
prep + cook time 25 minutes

750 g (1½ lb) potatoes, cubed
2 garlic cloves
6 tablespoons reduced-fat crème fraîche
1 tablespoon chopped sage
4 slices of calves' liver, about 150 g (5 oz) each
2 tablespoons seasoned flour
1 tablespoon olive oil
salt and pepper
gravy, to serve

1 Cook the potatoes and garlic in a saucepan of lightly salted boiling water for 10–12 minutes until tender, then drain.
2 Mash the potatoes and garlic with the crème fraîche and sage and season to taste with plenty of freshly ground black pepper.
3 Meanwhile, press the pieces of liver into the seasoned flour to coat them all over. Heat the oil in a nonstick frying pan, add the liver and fry for 1–2 minutes on each side or until cooked to your liking. Serve with the mash and gravy.

Tip
Liver is a good source of fat-soluble vitamin A, however you should avoid it if you are pregnant since excess vitamin A can be harmful to an unborn baby.

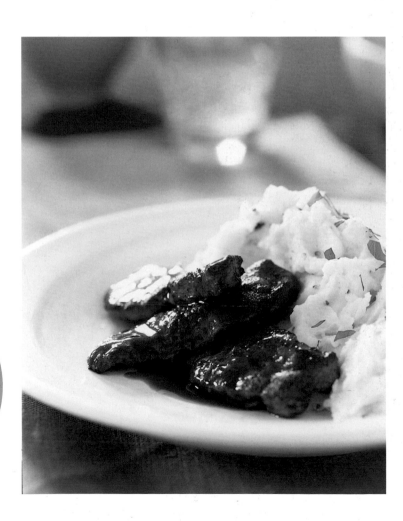

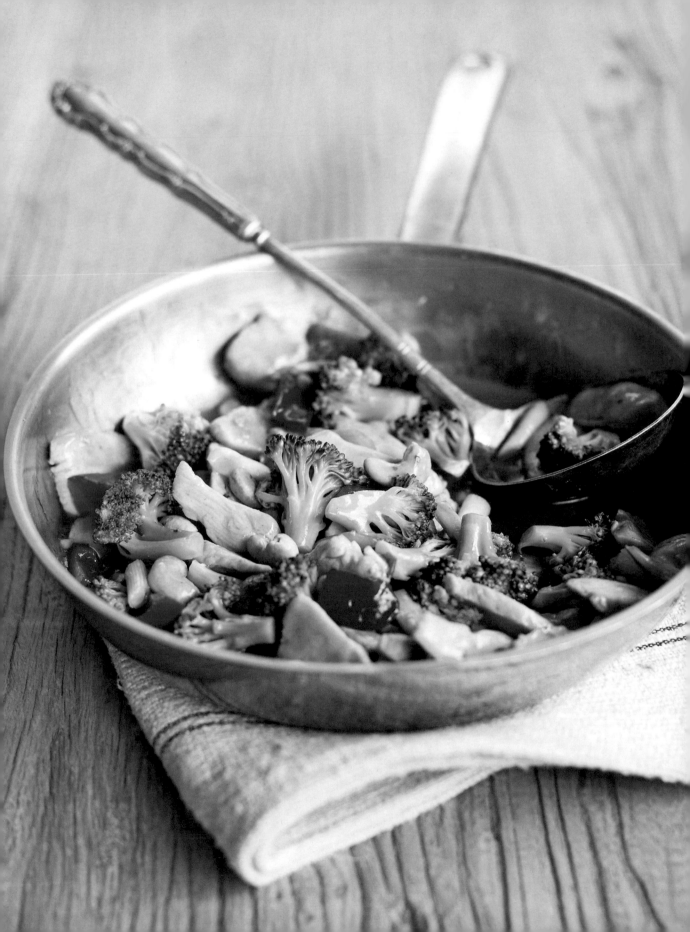

stir-fried lemon chicken with toasted cashews

serves 2
prep + cook time 20 minutes

1 tablespoon groundnut oil
250 (8 oz) skinless chicken
  breasts, sliced
125 g (4 oz) broccoli florets
1 small red pepper, roughly
  chopped
2 spring onions, thickly sliced
50 g (2 oz) unsalted cashew nuts
1 tablespoon cornflour
125 ml (4 fl oz) cold water
2 tablespoons lemon juice
1½ tablespoons honey
2 tablespoons light soy sauce
steamed rice or noodles, to serve
  (optional)

1 Heat the oil in a large wok or frying pan and cook the chicken for 3–4 minutes over a medium-high heat, until golden. Using a slotted spoon, transfer to a plate and set aside.
2 Return the pan to the heat and add the broccoli, red pepper and spring onions. Stir-fry for 3–4 minutes, until softened.
3 Meanwhile, place a small pan over a medium-low heat and toast the cashew nuts for 3–4 minutes, shaking the pan occasionally, until golden. Remove from the heat.
4 Dissolve the cornflour in a small bowl with 1 tablespoon of the water, then mix in the remaining water plus the lemon juice, honey and soy sauce. Add to the vegetables along with the cashew nuts. Reduce the heat to medium-low and return the chicken to the pan. Simmer for 2–3 minutes, until the chicken is cooked through and the sauce hot and thickened. Serve immediately, with steamed rice or noodles, if desired.

Tip
Although fairly calorific, cashews have high levels of iron, magnesium, phosphorus, zinc, copper and manganese and heart-healthy fatty acids.

herb pasta with roasted cherry tomatoes

serves 4
prep + cook time 25 minutes

375 g (12 oz) dried pasta shapes
200 g (7 oz) cherry tomatoes,
    halved
2 tablespoons pesto
1 tablespoon white wine vinegar
2 tablespoons capers, drained
2 anchovy fillets, chopped
    (optional)
2 tablespoons chopped mixed
    herbs, such as parsley and basil
salt and pepper
parmesan cheese shavings,
    to garnish
crisp green salad, to serve

1 Cook the pasta according to packet instructions and drain.
2 Meanwhile, place the tomatoes under a preheated hot grill and cook for about 15 minutes until they are slightly charred and beginning to dry out.
3 Place the pesto, vinegar, capers, anchovies and herbs in a food processor or blender and blend until almost smooth but retaining a little texture.
4 Toss the sauce through the hot pasta with the tomatoes, season to taste with salt and pepper and serve with some Parmesan shavings and a crisp green salad.

Tip
Pasta is a good staple for use in vegetarian meals as it is also a source of protein.

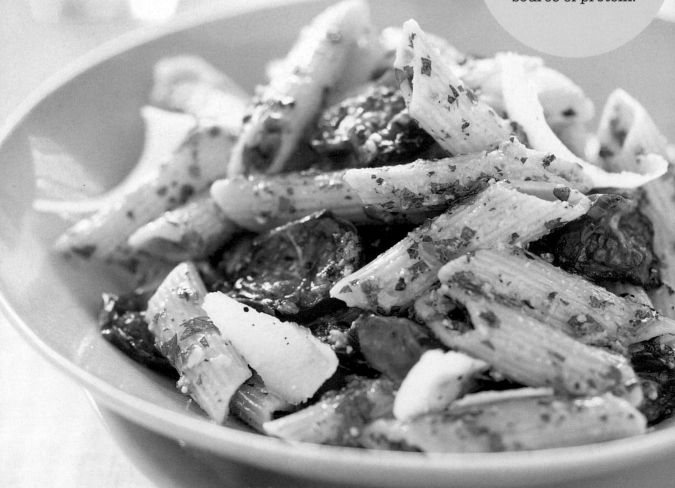

couscous with grilled vegetables

serves 4
prep + cook time 30 minutes

300 g (10 oz) couscous
500 ml (17 fl oz) boiling water
2 red peppers, cored, deseeded
   and quartered
1 orange pepper, cored, deseeded
   and quartered
6 baby courgettes, halved
   lengthways
2 red onions, cut into wedges
24 cherry tomatoes
2 garlic cloves, finely sliced
2 tablespoons olive oil
100 g (3½ oz) asparagus spears
grated rind and juice of 1 lemon
4 tablespoons chopped herbs
   (such as parsley or mint)
salt and pepper

1 Tip the couscous into a large bowl, pour over the water, cover and set aside for 10 minutes while preparing the remaining ingredients.
2 Place the peppers, courgettes, onions, tomatoes and garlic in a grill pan in one layer, drizzle over the oil and cook under a preheated hot grill for 5–6 minutes, turning the vegetables occasionally.
3 Add the asparagus to the pan and continue to grill for 2–3 minutes until the vegetables are tender and lightly charred. When they are cool enough to handle, remove the skins from the peppers and discard.
4 Fork through the couscous to separate the grains. Toss with the vegetables, lime rind and juice, and herbs, season to taste with salt and pepper and serve.

Tip
Cherry tomatoes are a good source of antioxidants, which help to improve general health and are thought to slow down the ageing process in the body.

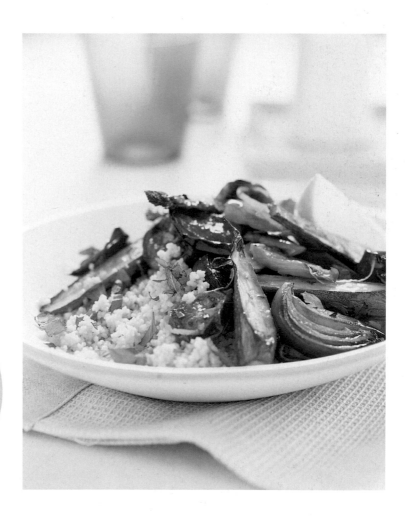

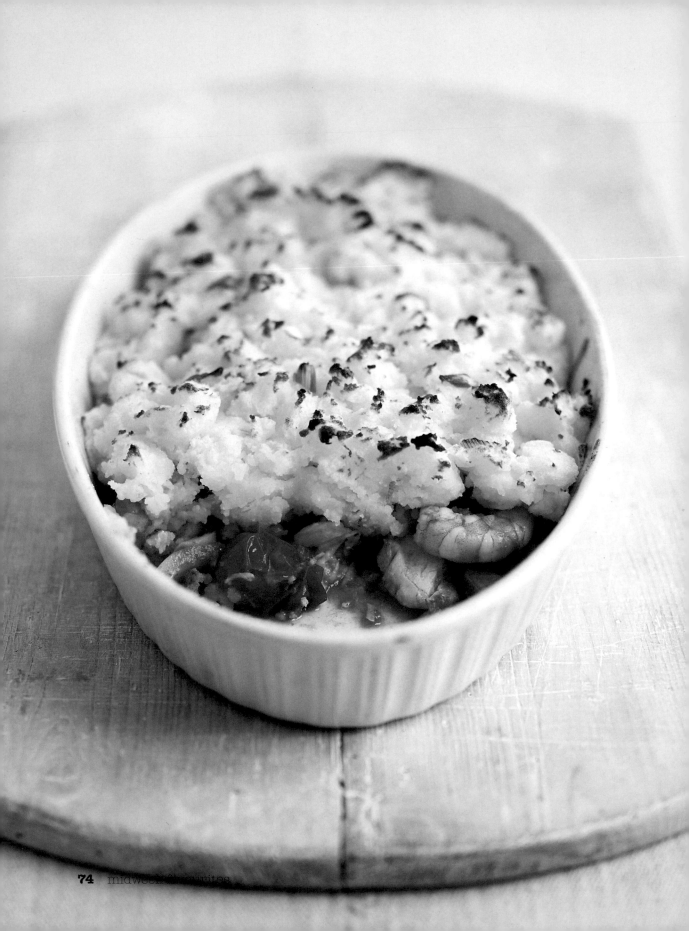

tomato & fennel fish pie

serves 4
prep + cook time 20 minutes

4 tablespoons olive oil
1 fennel bulb, chopped
2 garlic cloves, sliced
200 g (7 oz) cherry tomatoes
1 tablespoon tomato purée
50 ml (2 fl oz) dry white wine
75 ml (3 fl oz) water
300 g (10 oz) skinless cod fillets,
    cut into chunks
150 g (5 oz) raw peeled large
    prawns
750 g (1½ lb) potatoes, peeled
    and cut into chunks
2 spring onions, sliced
salt and pepper

1 Heat 1 tablespoon of the oil in a saucepan. Add the fennel and garlic and cook for 5–7 minutes until softened. Add the tomatoes and tomato purée and cook for a further 2 minutes until softened. Pour over the wine and cook until nearly boiled away, then add the measurement water and fish. Cook for 3 minutes. Add the prawns and cook for 3–5 minutes until just cooked through.

2 Meanwhile, cook the potatoes in a saucepan of lightly salted boiling water for 12–15 minutes until soft. Drain and mash with the remaining oil, the spring onions and a little water to loosen. Season well with salt and pepper.

3 Arrange the fish and sauce in a baking dish. Spoon over the mash. Cook under a preheated hot grill for 3 minutes until browned. Serve immediately.

caponata ratatouille

serves 6
prep + cook time 1 hour

750 g (1½ lb) aubergines
1 large onion
1 tablespoon olive oil
3 celery sticks, coarsely chopped
a little wine (optional)
2 large beef tomatoes, skinned
   and deseeded
1 teaspoon chopped thyme
¼–½ teaspoon cayenne pepper
2 tablespoons capers
handful of pitted green olives
4 tablespoons white wine vinegar
1 tablespoon sugar
1–2 tablespoons cocoa powder
   (optional)
freshly ground black pepper

to garnish
toasted, chopped almonds
chopped parsley

1 Cut the aubergines and onion into 1 cm (½ inch) chunks.
2 Heat the oil in a nonstick frying pan until very hot, add the aubergine and fry for about 15 minutes until very soft. Add a little boiling water to prevent sticking if necessary.
3 Meanwhile, place the onion and celery in a saucepan with a little water or wine. Cook for 5 minutes until tender but still firm.
4 Add the tomatoes, thyme, cayenne pepper and aubergine and onions. Cook for 15 minutes, stirring occasionally. Add the capers, olives, wine vinegar, sugar and cocoa powder (if using) and cook for 2–3 minutes.
5 Season with pepper and serve garnished with almonds and parsley. Serve hot or cold as a side dish, starter or a main dish, with polenta and hot crusty bread, if liked.

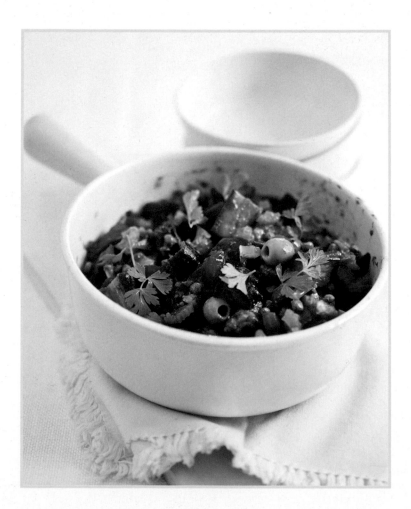

zingy wild mushroom rice

serves 4
prep + cook time 30 minutes

25 g (1 oz) butter
1 tablespoon olive oil
200 g (7 oz) wild mushrooms,
    roughly chopped
1 onion, finely chopped
2 garlic cloves, crushed
250 g (8 oz) mixed wild and
    basmati rice
750 ml (1¼ pints) vegetable stock
finely grated rind and juice of
    1 lemon
2 spring onions, chopped
large handful of chopped parsley
½ red chilli, chopped
salt and pepper

1 Heat the butter and oil in a large, heavy-based saucepan. Add the mushrooms and cook for 3 minutes until golden, then remove from the pan and set aside. Add the onion to the pan and cook for 5 minutes until softened, then stir in the garlic. Add the rice and stir until coated in the oil, then pour in the stock.

2 Bring to the boil, then reduce the heat and simmer for about 15 minutes until most of the liquid has been absorbed. Return the mushrooms to the pan, cover and cook very gently for 5–7 minutes until the rice is tender. Season to taste and stir in the remaining ingredients before serving.

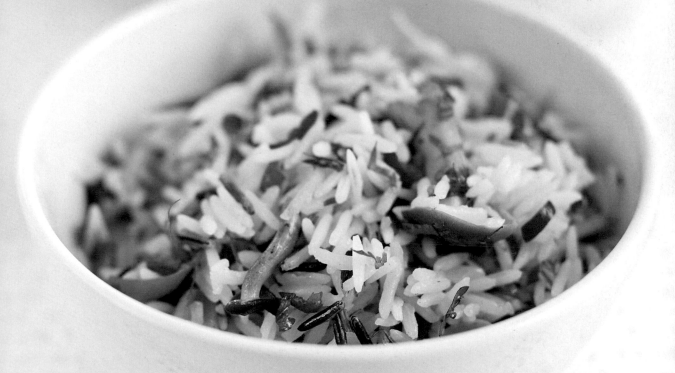

spicy chickpea curry

serves 4
prep + cook time 30 minutes

2 tablespoons sunflower oil
4 garlic cloves, minced
2 teaspoons peeled and finely
   grated fresh root ginger
1 large onion, coarsely grated
1–2 green chillies, finely sliced
1 teaspoon hot chilli powder
1 tablespoon ground cumin
1 tablespoon ground coriander
3 tablespoons reduced-fat natural
   yogurt, plus extra, whisked, to
   serve
2 teaspoons garam masala
500 ml (17 fl oz) water
2 teaspoons tamarind paste
2 teaspoons medium or hot curry
   powder
2 x 400 g (13 oz) cans chickpeas,
   rinsed and drained
chopped coriander leaves,
   to garnish
lemon wedges, to serve (optional)

1 Heat the oil in a large heavy-based frying pan, add the garlic, ginger, onion and green chillies and cook over a medium heat, stirring occasionally, for 5–6 minutes until the onion is lightly golden. Add the chilli powder, cumin, ground coriander, yogurt and garam masala and cook for a further 1–2 minutes.

2 Stir in the measurement water and bring to the boil. Add the tamarind paste, curry powder and chickpeas and bring back to the boil, then reduce the heat to medium and cook, uncovered, for 15–20 minutes or until the sauce is thickened.

3 Ladle into bowls, drizzle with extra whisked yogurt and scatter with chopped coriander. Serve with lemon wedges for squeezing over, if liked.

Tip
Garam masala is a classic Indian spice mix. Recipes for it vary, but it usually comprises ground cardamom, cloves, cumin, cinnamon, peppercorns and nutmeg.

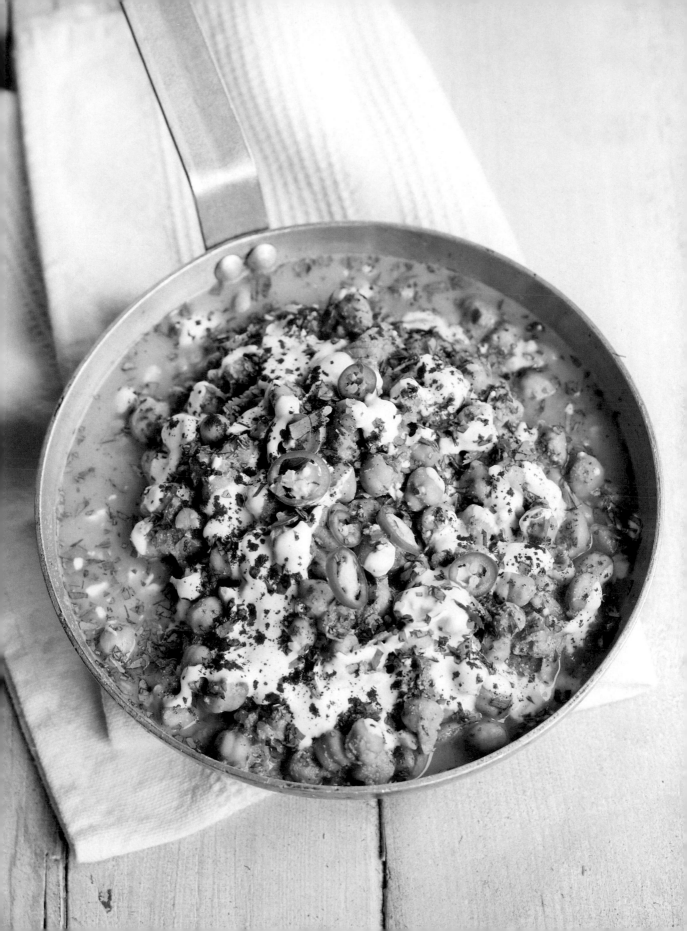

herby lentils with parma ham crisps

serves 4
prep + cook time 15 minutes

2 tablespoons olive oil
1 garlic clove, crushed
4 spring onions, sliced
2 x 400 g (13 oz) cans green lentils,
   drained and rinsed
2 tablespoons balsamic vinegar
3 tablespoons chopped herbs,
   such as parsley, oregano or basil
125 g (4 oz) cherry tomatoes,
   halved
85 g (3¼ oz) sliced Parma ham

1 Heat the oil in a nonstick saucepan, add the garlic and spring onions and fry for 2 minutes.
2 Stir in the lentils, vinegar, herbs and tomatoes and set aside.
3 Heat a frying pan until hot, add the Parma ham and cook for 1–2 minutes, until crisp. Arrange the lentil salad on a large serving dish, place the ham on top and serve.

Tip
Lentils are a good source of protein and iron, as well as containing isoflavones which may relieve menopausal symptoms.

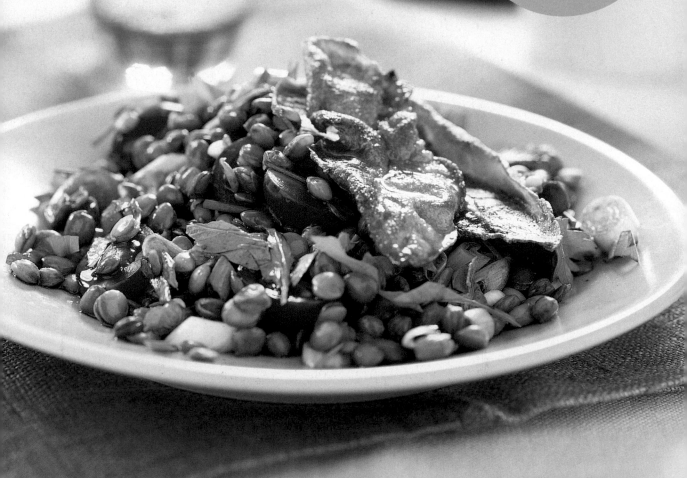

pasta with prawns, peas & mint

serves 4
prep + cook time 25 minutes

375 g (12 oz) dried pasta shapes
200 g (7 oz) frozen peas
1 tablespoon olive oil
1 onion, sliced
1 garlic clove, crushed
150 ml (¼ pint) dry white wine
200 g (7 oz) cooked tiger prawns
6 tablespoons reduced-fat crème
   fraîche
2 tablespoons freshly grated
   Parmesan cheese
2 tablespoons chopped mint
salt and pepper
mint leaves, to garnish

1 Cook the pasta according to packet instructions, adding the peas 2 minutes before the end of cooking time. Drain.
2 Meanwhile, heat the oil in a nonstick saucepan, add the onion and garlic and fry for 2–3 minutes until they begin to soften.
3 Add the wine to the pan, bring to the boil and boil until reduced by about a half.
4 Stir in the prawns, crème fraîche, Parmesan and mint and heat through. Season to taste with salt and pepper. Toss the sauce through the pasta and serve garnished with mint leaves.

Tip
Although shellfish are a source of cholesterol they can be included in your diet as blood cholesterol is more affected by the amount of saturated fat in a diet and other factors such as weight.

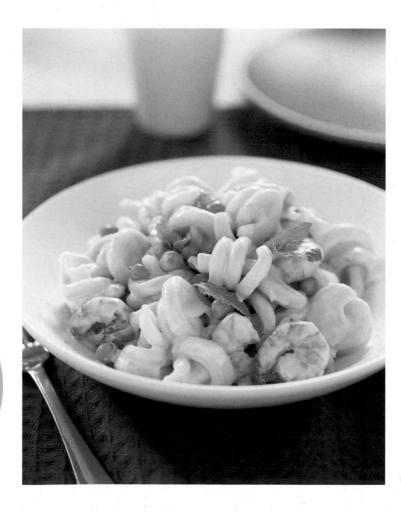

crispy salmon ramen

serves 2
prep + cook time 20 minutes

2 teaspoons groundnut oil
2 boneless salmon fillets, skin on
500 ml (17 fl oz) hot clear
   chicken stock
1 tablespoon lime juice
2 teaspoons fish sauce
1 tablespoon light soy sauce
1.5 cm (¾ inch) piece of fresh
   root ginger, peeled and cut
   into matchsticks
1 small red chilli, thinly sliced
2 heads of pak choi, sliced in half
   lengthways
150 g (5 oz) ramen or egg noodles
coriander leaves, to garnish

1 Place the oil in a large frying pan over a medium heat and fry the salmon fillets, skin-side down, for 3–5 minutes, until the skin is really crispy. Turn carefully and cook for a further minute, until still slightly rare. Transfer to a plate and keep warm.

2 Pour the stock into a saucepan, add the lime juice, fish sauce, soy sauce and ginger and bring to the boil. Simmer for 3–4 minutes, then add the chilli and pak choi and simmer for another 4–5 minutes, until tender.

3 Meanwhile, cook the noodles in a pan of boiling water for 2–3 minutes, or according to the packet instructions, until just tender. Drain and heap into bowls.

4 Ladle over the hot broth and top each bowl with a salmon fillet. Serve immediately, garnished with coriander leaves.

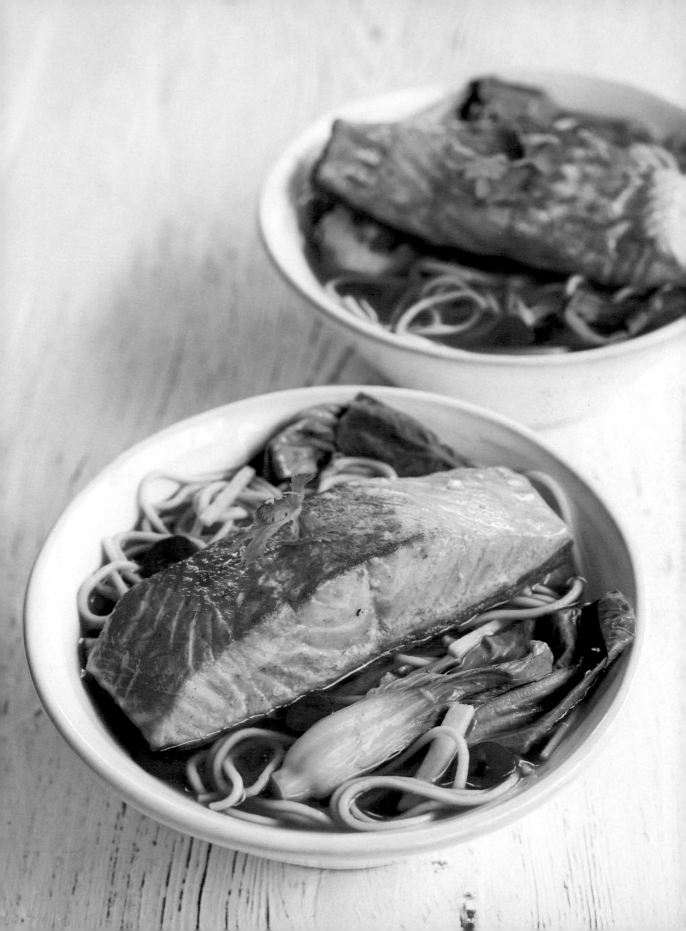

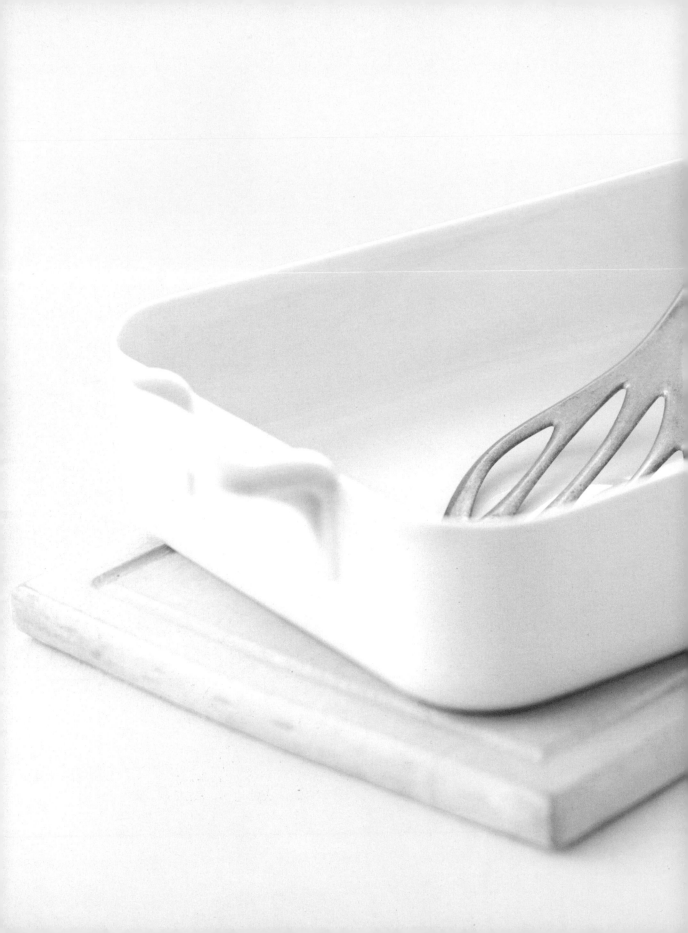

food for friends

pork, apple & ginger stir-fry

serves 4
prep + cook time 20 minutes

2 tablespoons sesame seeds
1 tablespoon coconut oil
300 g (10 oz) pork fillet, in strips
2 garlic cloves, chopped
5-cm (2-inch) fresh root ginger,
    peeled and cut into matchsticks
1 green chilli, deseeded and
    chopped
2 apples, cored and cut into
    wedges
2 carrots, cut into matchsticks
150 g (5 oz) broccoli florets
300 g (10 oz) ribbon rice noodles
juice of 1 lime

1 Heat a nonstick frying pan over a medium-low heat and dry-fry the sesame seeds for 2 minutes, stirring frequently, until golden and toasted. Set aside.

2 Heat the oil in a wok or large frying pan, add the pork and stir-fry for 6–8 minutes until lightly browned. Add the garlic, ginger, chilli, apples and vegetables and stir-fry for a further 4–5 minutes or until the pork is cooked through.

3 Meanwhile, cook the noodles according to the pack instructions, then add to the stir-fry with the lime juice and toss all the ingredients together.

4 Serve sprinkled with the toasted sesame seeds.

Tip
Coconut oil gives a delicious sweet undernote to curries and stir-fries but it is high in fat so make sure you use just a little.

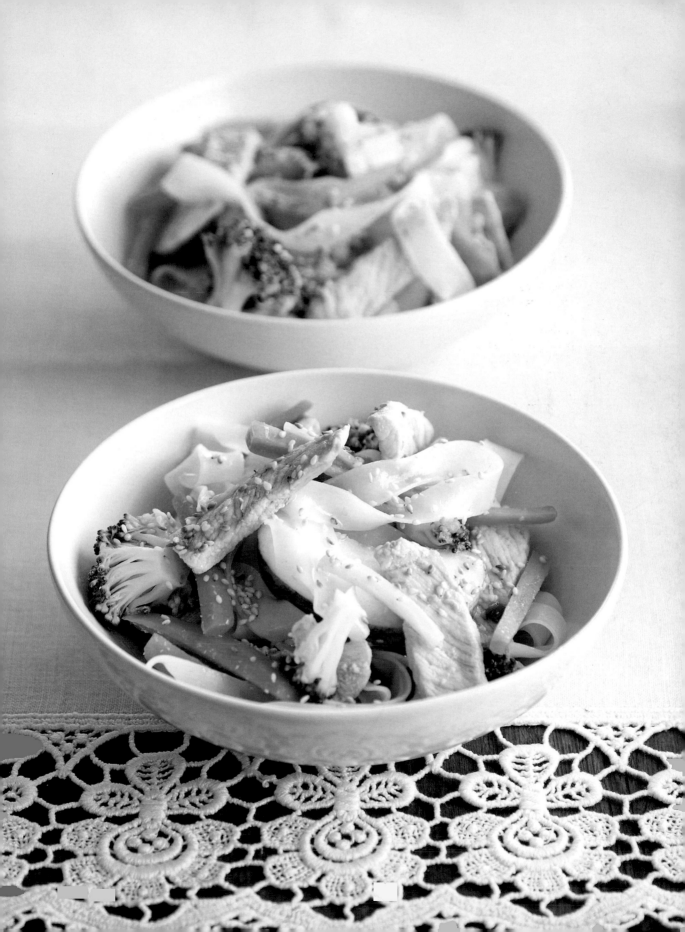

lemon & garlic chicken breasts with rosemary gravy

serves 4
prep + cook time 30 minutes

4 chicken breasts, each about
    150 g (5 oz) (with skin on)
1 lemon, sliced
4 rosemary sprigs
8 garlic cloves, peeled
2 tablespoons olive oil
salt and pepper

for the gravy
1 tablespoon olive oil
1 tablespoon chopped rosemary
    leaves
300 ml (½ pint) chicken stock
6 tablespoons white wine
2 teaspoons cornflour

to serve
green beans
boiled potatoes

1 Make a large slit in the side of each chicken breast and insert 2 slices of lemon, 1 rosemary sprig and a halved garlic clove. Tie each chicken with with string around the centre, then put the chicken in a roasting tin, drizzle with olive oil and season generously with salt and pepper. Roast in a preheated oven, 220°C (425°F), Gas Mark 7, for 20–25 minutes or until golden and cooked through.

2 Meanwhile, make the gravy. Heat the oil in a small saucepan and cook the rosemary leaves for 1 minute over a moderate heat. Pour in the stock and wine and bring to the boil. Continue to boil for 5 minutes to infuse the flavours and reduce a little. Blend the cornflour with 2 tablespoons water and add to the gravy, stirring continually to thicken. Pour over the roasted chicken pieces and serve with green beans and boiled potatoes.

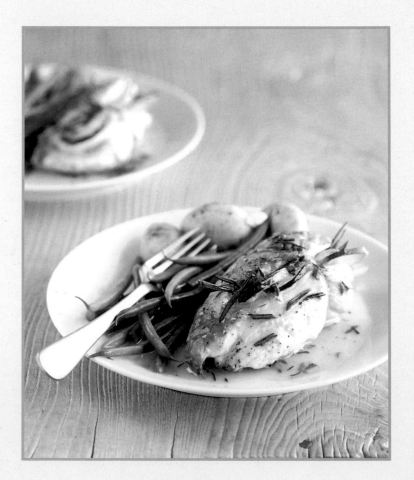

chicken with spinach & ricotta

serves 4
prep + cook time 30 minutes

4 boneless, skinless chicken
   breasts, 125 g (4 oz) each
125 g (4 oz) ricotta cheese
125 g (4 oz) cooked spinach,
   squeezed dry
¼ teaspoon grated nutmeg
8 slices Parma ham
2 tablespoons olive oil, plus extra
   for drizzling
salt and pepper

to serve
lemon wedges
rocket leaves

1 Make a long horizontal slit through the thickest part of each chicken breast without cutting right through.

2 Crumble the ricotta into a bowl. Chop the spinach and mix into the ricotta with the nutmeg. Season with salt and pepper.

3 Divide the stuffing between the slits in the chicken breasts and wrap each one in 2 pieces of Parma ham, winding it around the chicken to cover the meat totally.

4 Heat the oil in a shallow ovenproof pan, add the chicken breasts and sauté for 4 minutes on each side or until the ham starts to brown. Transfer to a preheated oven, 200°C (400°F), Gas Mark 6, and cook for 15 minutes. Serve with lemon wedges and rocket leaves drizzled with olive oil.

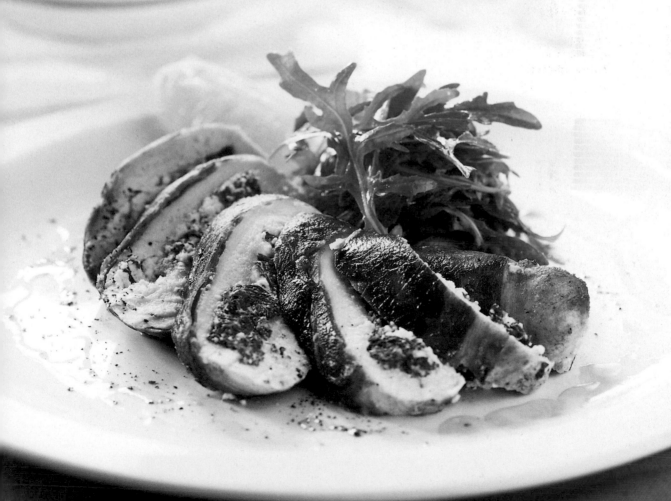

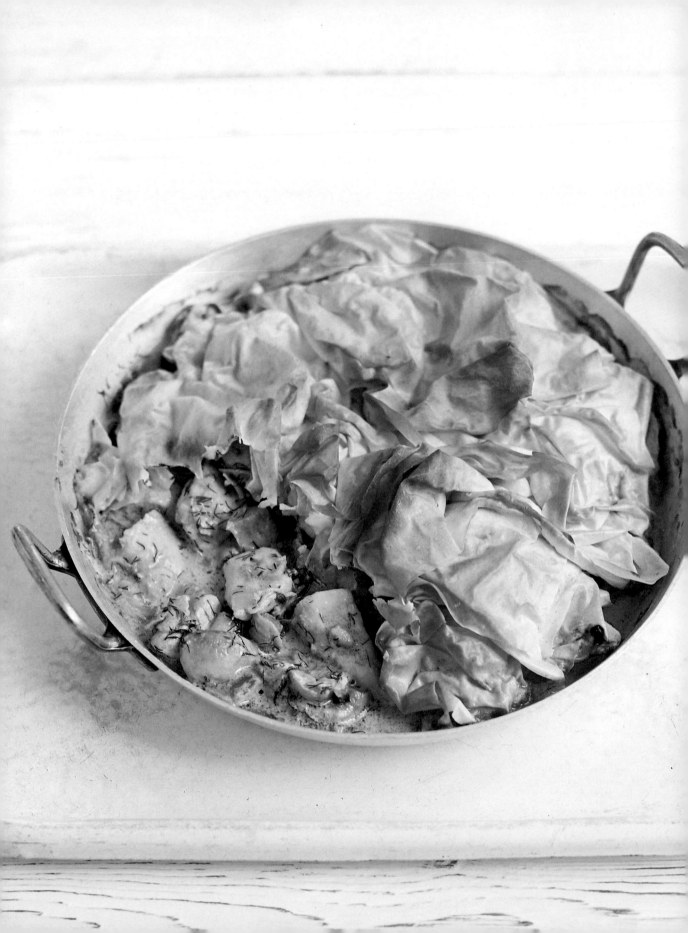

filo-topped chicken, mushroom & dill pie

serves 4
prep + cook time 30 minutes

1 tablespoon vegetable oil
1 onion, finely chopped
300 g (10 oz) skinless chicken
    breast fillets, diced
150 g (5 oz) mushrooms, halved
    if large
3 tablespoons dry white wine
5 tablespoons reduced-fat crème
    fraîche
finely grated rind of 1 lemon
handful of chopped dill
3 large filo pastry sheets
40 g (1½ oz) butter, melted
salt and pepper

1 Heat the oil in a shallow, ovenproof casserole dish. Add the onion and cook for 2 minutes, then stir in the chicken and cook for a further 5 minutes. Add the mushrooms and continue to cook for 1 minute until starting to soften.

2 Pour in the wine, cook until it has bubbled away, then stir in the crème fraîche, lemon rind and dill and remove from the heat. Season to taste.

3 Meanwhile, unwrap the filo pastry and cover with a piece of damp kitchen paper until ready to use it. Working quickly, brush 1 sheet with melted butter and cut into 3 long strips. Arrange the strips on top of the chicken, scrunching it up a little. Repeat with the remaining pastry until the chicken is covered.

4 Brush all over with any remaining butter, then place in a preheated oven, 200°C (400°F), Gas Mark 6, for 15–20 minutes until the filo pastry is crisp and the chicken is cooked through.

Tip
Using delicate filo pastry is easy but you need to keep it covered with a damp tea towel, kitchen roll or its plastic wrap to stop it drying out.

roast chicken with spice rub

serves 4
prep + cook time 1 hour 40 minutes
to 1 hour 50 minutes

1.5 kg (3 lb) whole chicken
3 tablespoons olive oil
1 teaspoon fennel seeds, roughly
    crushed
1 teaspoon cumin seeds, roughly
    crushed
1 teaspoon crushed dried red
    chillies
1 teaspoon dried oregano
½ teaspoon ground cinnamon
625 g (1¼ lb) baby new potatoes
2 shallots, finely chopped
2 garlic cloves, finely chopped
    (optional)
150 g (5 oz) fine green beans
juice of 1 lemon
200 ml (7 fl oz) chicken stock
small bunch fresh coriander or
    flat leaf parsley, or mix of the
    two, roughly chopped
salt and pepper

1 Put the chicken into a large roasting tin. Drizzle with 2 tablespoons of the oil. Mix the crushed seeds, chillies, oregano and cinnamon with some salt and pepper, then sprinkle half over the chicken.

2 Cover the chicken loosely with foil, then roast in a preheated oven, 190°C (375°F), Gas Mark 5, for 40 minutes. Remove the foil and baste with the pan juices. Add the potatoes to the tin, toss in the juices, then cook uncovered for 40–50 minutes, basting and turning the potatoes once or twice until golden brown. Re-cover the chicken with foil if the spice rub begins to overbrown.

3 Meanwhile, heat the remaining oil in a small saucepan, add the shallots and garlic, if liked, and fry for 5 minutes until softened. Stir in the remaining spice rub and cook for 1 minute. Cook the green beans in a saucepan of boiling water for 5 minutes, then drain and toss in the shallot mixture with the lemon juice.

4 When the chicken is cooked, add the green-bean mixture to the potatoes. Mix together, then add the stock and bring to the boil on the hob. Sprinkle with the herbs, carve the chicken and serve.

Tip
The baby new potatoes used in this spicy all-in-one dish are medium GI and so are a good choice for steady blood glucose levels.

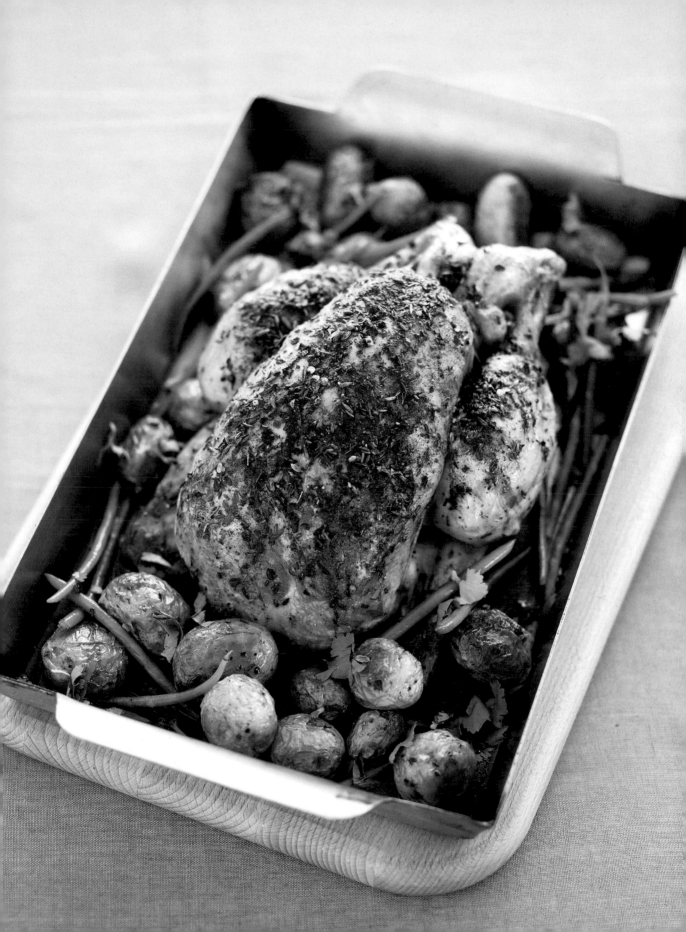

lamb fillet with beetroot salad

serves 4
prep + cook time 25 minutes

125 g (4 oz) Puy lentils
125 g (4 oz) fine green beans
4 tablespoons extra virgin olive oil
2 best end of neck fillets or lamb
    loins, about 300 g (10 oz) each
4 tablespoons red wine
1 tablespoon red wine vinegar
375 g (12 oz) cooked beetroot in
    natural juices, drained and diced
1 small bunch of mint, roughly
    chopped
salt and pepper

1 Put the lentils into a saucepan, cover with cold water and simmer for 20 minutes. Drain well and transfer to a bowl.
2 Meanwhile, cook the green beans in lightly salted boiling water for 2–3 minutes, then plunge immediately into a bowl of ice-cold water. This is known as blanching. Drain and pat dry on kitchen paper.
3 Heat 1 tablespoon of the oil in a frying pan and fry the lamb fillets for 7 minutes, turning once. Transfer to a low oven, 150°C (300°F), Gas Mark 2, to rest for 5 minutes, reserving the juices in the pan.
4 Add the wine to the pan juices and boil until only about 1 tablespoon remains. Remove from the heat and whisk in the vinegar and the remaining oil and season to taste with salt and pepper.
5 Combine the lentils, beans, beetroot and mint in a bowl, add the dressing and toss to coat. Serve with the lamb.

Tip
Puy lentils have a delicious peppery flavour and hold their shape well when cooked, unlike most lentils. They contain vitamins A, C and dietary fibre.

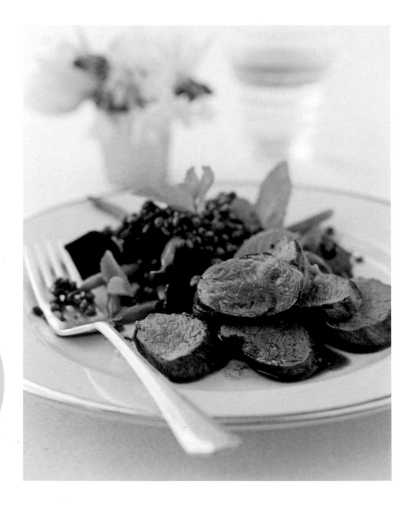

fragrant vietnamese beef curry

serves 4
prep + cook time 35–40 minutes

2 tablespoons groundnut oil
750 g (1½ lb) thin-cut fillet steak,
  cut into strips
1 onion, finely sliced
4 garlic cloves, crushed
1 fresh red chilli, finely sliced
2 star anise
1 teaspoon cardamom seeds,
  crushed
1 cinnamon stick
300 g (10 oz) French beans,
  trimmed
1 carrot, cut into batons
2 tablespoons Thai fish sauce
2 tablespoons ground bean sauce

to garnish
small handful of finely chopped
  coriander leaves
small handful of finely chopped
  mint leaves

1 Heat half the oil in a large nonstick frying pan and stir-fry the beef in batches for 1–2 minutes. Remove with a slotted spoon and keep warm.

2 Heat the remaining oil in the frying pan and stir-fry the onion for 4–5 minutes until softened, then add the garlic, chilli, star anise, cardamom, cinnamon, beans and carrot. Stir-fry for 6–8 minutes.

3 Return the beef to the pan with the fish sauce and ground bean sauce. Stir-fry for 3–4 minutes or until heated through. Remove from the heat and sprinkle over the chopped herbs just before serving.

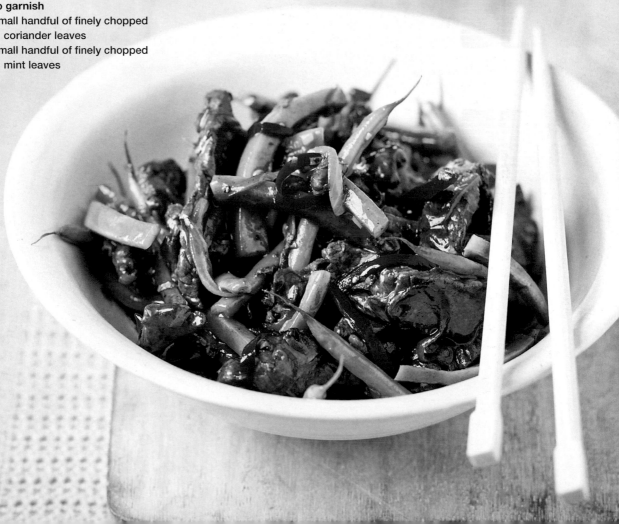

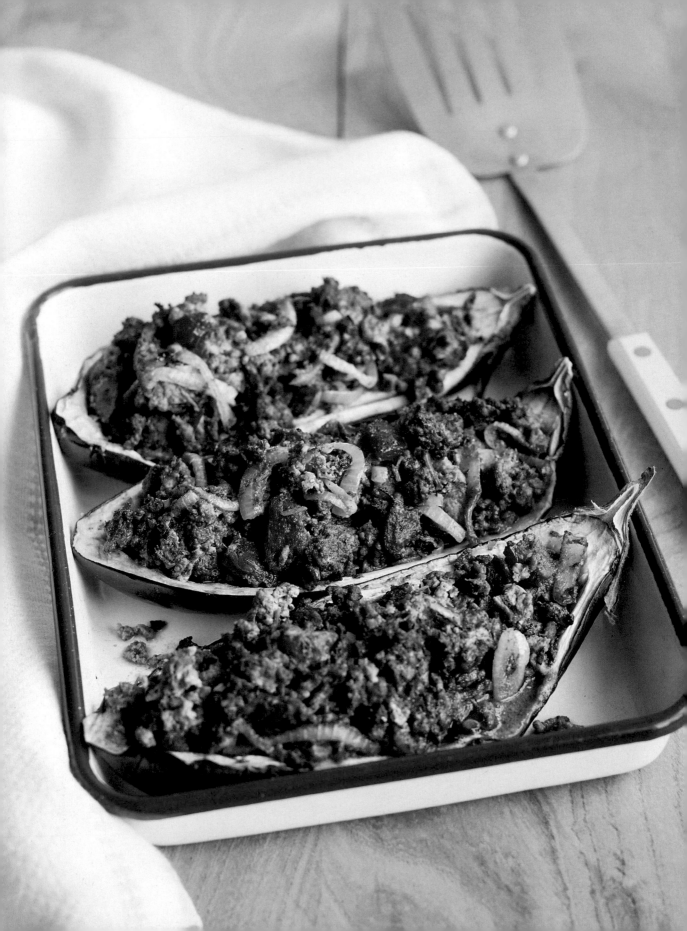

spicy lamb-stuffed aubergines

serves 4
prep + cook time 1 hour

2 large aubergines
1 tablespoon groundnut oil
1 onion, thinly sliced
1 teaspoon peeled and finely
    grated fresh root ginger
1 teaspoon hot chilli powder
1 tablespoon medium curry paste
2 garlic cloves, crushed
¼ teaspoon ground turmeric
1 teaspoon ground coriander
2 teaspoons dried mint
1 ripe tomato, finely chopped
500 g (1 lb) lean minced lamb
100 g (3½ oz) roasted red peppers
    in brine, drained and finely diced
2 tablespoons chopped coriander
    leaves
2 tablespoons chopped mint
    leaves
salt

1 Preheat the oven to 180°C (350°F), Gas Mark 4. Cut the aubergines in half lengthways, use a spoon to scoop out most of the flesh and discard it. Place the aubergines, cut sides up, on a baking sheet and set aside.

2 Heat the oil in a large frying pan over a medium heat. Add the onion and stir-fry for 4–5 minutes until soft. Now add the ginger, chilli powder, curry paste, garlic, turmeric, ground coriander, dried mint and chopped tomato, and stir-fry for 4–5 minutes. Season to taste.

3 Add the lamb and continue to stir-fry for 5–6 minutes over a high heat until well browned. Stir in the red pepper and herbs and mix well. Spoon the lamb mixture into the prepared aubergine shells and cook in the preheated oven for 20–25 minutes. Serve immediately with a herby tabbouleh.

Tip
The ginger and turmeric used in this lamb dish both contain powerful anti-inflammatory compounds for an additional health boost.

kale & pecorino pesto linguini

serves 4
prep + cook time 30 minutes

375 g (12 oz) linguini
300 g (10 oz) kale
2 tablespoons olive oil
3 garlic cloves, crushed
100 g (3½ oz) toasted pine nuts
100 g (3½ oz) mascarpone cheese
100 g (3½ oz) pecorino cheese,
    grated, plus extra shavings
    to garnish
½ teaspoon grated nutmeg
salt and pepper

1 Cook the pasta according to the packet instructions.

2 Meanwhile, wash the kale well, remove any tough stems and chop roughly.

3 Heat the oil in a pan and sauté the garlic for 2–3 minutes. Add the kale to the pan. Cover and cook for 2–3 minutes, or until the kale starts to wilt.

4 Place the pine nuts into a food processor or blender and whizz until smooth. Tip in the mascarpone, pecorino and nutmeg. Whizz again.

5 Add the kale and garlic mixture and whizz until smooth. Season to taste.

6 Drain the pasta and return it to the pan. Add the pesto and toss to mix well. Serve garnished with shavings of pecorino.

Tip
This unusual take on pesto uses nutritional power food kale. One cup of kale provides over 100 per cent of your recommended daily allowance of vitamins K and C.

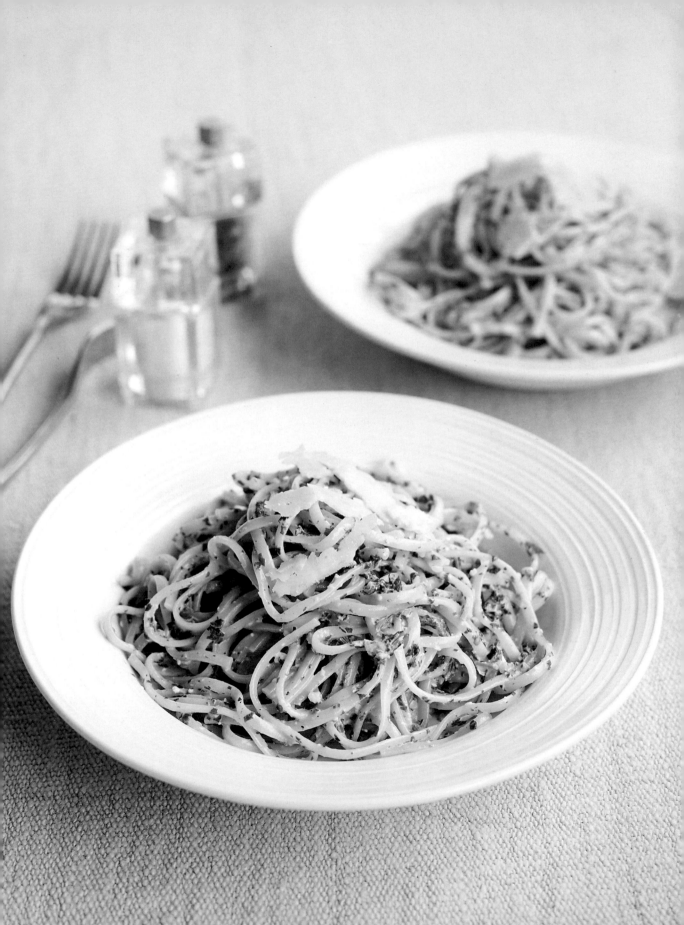

smoked salmon & cream cheese risotto

serves 4
prep + cook time 35 minutes

2 teaspoons olive oil
1 onion, finely chopped
2 garlic cloves, crushed
300 g (10 oz) risotto rice
150 ml (¼ pint) dry white wine
900 ml (1½ pints) simmering
   vegetable stock
125 g (4 oz) reduced-fat cream
   cheese
125 g (4 oz) smoked salmon,
   chopped
4 tablespoons chopped herbs,
   such as chives, parsley or dill
salt and pepper

1 Heat the oil in a large saucepan, add the onion and garlic and fry for 2–3 minutes until they begin to soften.
2 Stir in the rice and continue to cook for 1 minute. Add the wine and cook, stirring, until all the wine has been absorbed.
3 Reduce the heat and add the stock a little at a time, stirring continuously, and allowing each amount of stock to be absorbed before adding the next. Continue until all the stock has been absorbed.
4 Stir in the cream cheese, smoked salmon and herbs, season to taste with salt and pepper and serve.

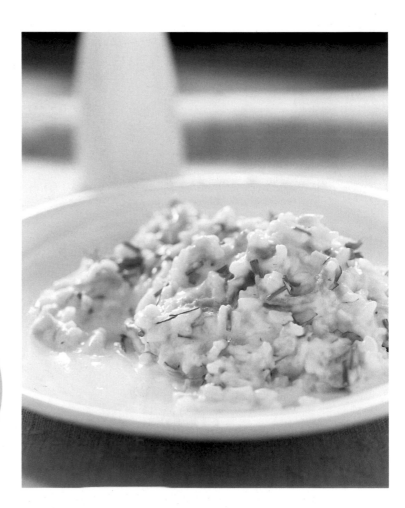

Tip
Smoked salmon is an oily fish which contains omega-3 fatty acids, which help to protect against heart disease. Try to eat oily fish at least once a week.

plaice florentine

serves 4
prep + cook time 20 minutes

15 g (½ oz) butter, plus extra for
    greasing
1 tablespoon plain flour
150 ml (¼ pint) semi-skimmed milk
50 g (2 oz) reduced-fat Cheddar
    cheese, grated
150 g (5 oz) frozen spinach
2 large plaice fillets, about 175 g
    (6 oz) each, halved to make
    4 thin fillets
25 g (1 oz) Parmesan cheese,
    grated
salt and pepper
mashed potato, to serve

1 Melt the butter in a saucepan. Stir in the flour and cook for
2 minutes. Slowly whisk in the milk until smooth. Bring to the boil,
whisking, then simmer for a few minutes until thickened. Take off
the heat, stir in the cheese and season.
2 Place the spinach in a sieve and pour over boiling water until
thawed. Drain well, then roughly chop. Place the fish on a lightly
greased baking sheet. Spread a layer of spinach on top of each fillet,
then drizzle over some of the white sauce. Sprinkle with the Parmesan.
3 Place in a preheated oven, 200°C (400°F), Gas Mark 6, for
10–12 minutes until the fish is just cooked through. Serve immediately
with mashed potato.

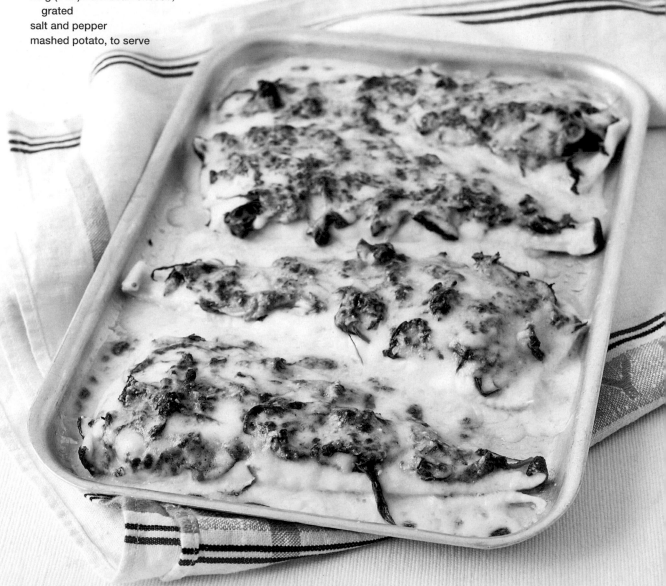

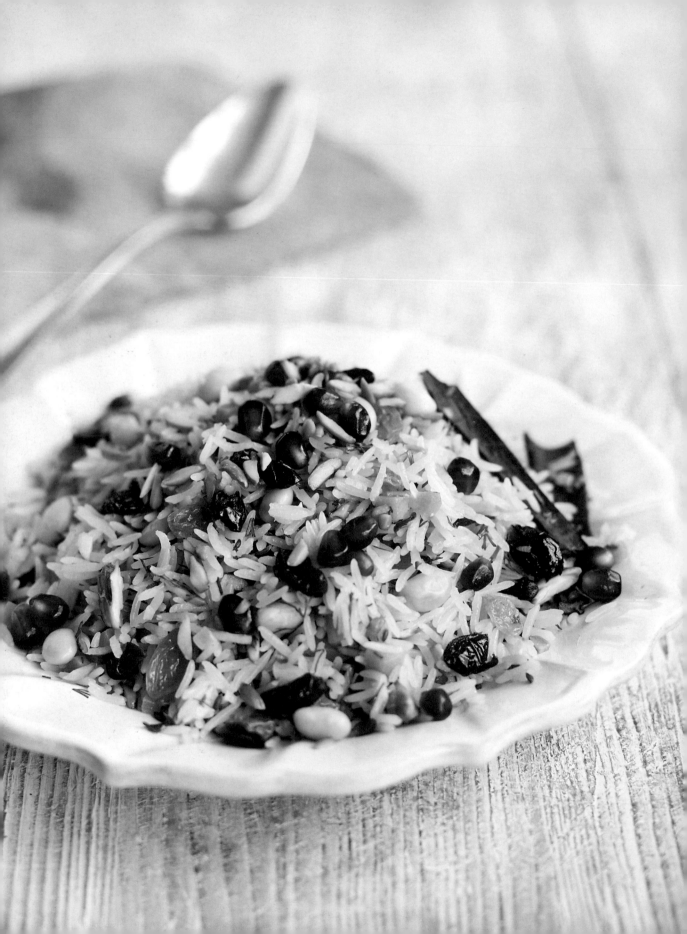

jewelled fruity spicy pilaf

serves 4
prep + cook time 30 minutes

1 tablespoon saffron threads
1 litre (1¾ pints) hot vegetable
 stock
400 g (13 oz) basmati rice
1 tablespoon olive oil
1 tablespoon butter
3 shallots, finely chopped
2 cloves garlic, finely chopped
4 cardamom pods, lightly bruised
2 cloves
2 cinnamon sticks
2 teaspoons cumin seeds
2 carrots, peeled and finely diced
4 tablespoons chopped dill
300 g (10 oz) podded soya beans
100 g (3½ oz) golden sultanas
100 g (3½ oz) dried cranberries
seeds from 1 ripe pomegranate
50 g (2 oz) slivered pistachio nuts
salt and pepper

1 Add the saffron to the hot stock and set aside.
2 Rinse the rice in cold running water and leave to drain.
3 Heat the oil and butter in a heavy-based saucepan and stir-fry the shallots and garlic for 1–2 minutes over a medium heat.
4 Add the cardamom pods, cloves, cinnamon sticks, cumin seeds, rice and carrots and stir to mix well. Add the stock mixture along with the dill, season and bring up to the boil. Then stir in the soya beans, golden sultanas and dried cranberries. Cover tightly and reduce the heat to low. Cook for 10–12 minutes without lifting the lid.
5 Remove from the heat and allow to stand, undisturbed, for 10 minutes.
6 Remove the lid (the liquid should have been completely absorbed), stir in the pomegranate seeds and pistachio nuts and serve immediately.

Tip
Basmati rice is digested slowly and releases sugar more slowly into the blood than many types of rice, so is an excellent choice for diabetes.

chilli spaghetti vongole

serves 4
prep + cook time 20 minutes

450 g (14½ oz) dried spaghetti
6 tablespoons extra-virgin olive oil,
   plus extra to serve
2 garlic cloves, chopped
2 red chillies, deseeded and finely
   chopped
4 anchovy fillets in oil, drained
   and chopped
small handful of flat leaf parsley,
   finely chopped
1 kg (2¼ lb) fresh clams, scrubbed
100 ml (3½ fl oz) dry white wine
salt and pepper

1 Cook the pasta in a large saucepan of lightly salted boiling water according to the packet instructions until al dente. Drain, then return to the pan.
2 Meanwhile, heat the oil in a frying pan, add the garlic, red chillies, anchovies and half the parsley and fry gently for a couple of minutes. Add the clams to the pan, discarding any that are cracked or don't shut when tapped. Pour in the wine, then increase the heat to high, cover tightly and cook for 4–5 minutes or until the clams have opened. Discard any that remain closed.
3 Add the clams and the juices to the spaghetti with the remaining parsley, then season and toss to mix well. Divide into bowls, drizzle with a little extra olive oil and serve immediately.

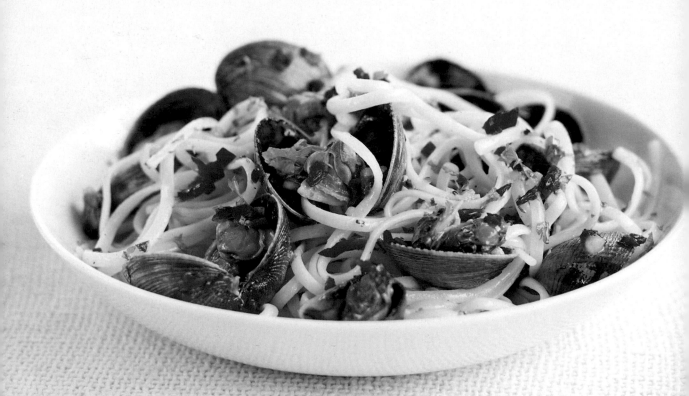

lemon sole with spicy salsa

serves 4
prep + cook time 20 minutes

4 lemon sole fillets, 225 g (7½ oz)
    each, skinned
salt and pepper

salsa
1 ripe mango, peeled, stoned and
    finely diced
1 red pepper, cored, deseeded
    and finely chopped
100 g (3½ oz) cherry tomatoes,
    quartered
1 red onion, finely chopped
½ teaspoon caster sugar
1 red chilli, deseeded and finely
    chopped
4 tablespoons chopped coriander
    leaves, plus extra to garnish
2 tablespoons rice vinegar
finely grated rind and juice of
    1 lime
1 teaspoon chilli oil
2 tablespoons olive oil

to serve
lime wedges
steamed basmati rice

1 To make the salsa, mix together all the ingredients in a large bowl and season well.

2 Place the fish fillets on a clean work surface, skinned-side up, and cut into half lengthways. Spoon some of the salsa on to the tail ends of the fish, roll up tightly, then season and place in a large nonstick frying pan. Cover and cook over a low heat for 8–10 minutes. Remove the lid and cook, uncovered, for a further 3 minutes or until cooked through.

3 Transfer the fish on to serving plates and scatter with chopped coriander. Serve with the remaining salsa, lime wedges to squeeze over and steamed basmati rice.

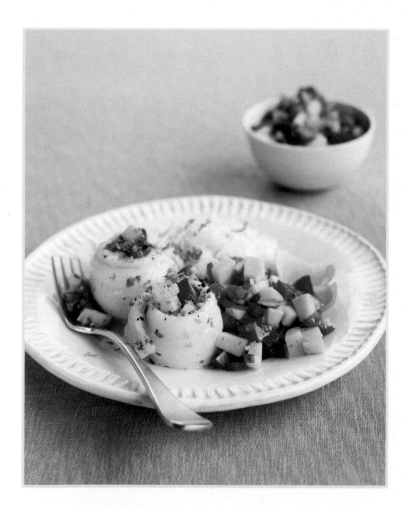

baked mushroom risotto

serves 4
prep + cook time 1 hour 30 minutes

30 g (1½ oz) dried porcini
   mushrooms, soaked in
   125 ml (4 fl oz) boiling water
   for 10–15 minutes
25 g (1 oz) butter
1 tablespoon olive oil
2 shallots, finely chopped
1 leek, trimmed, cleaned and finely
   chopped
1 large garlic clove, finely chopped
350 g (11½ oz) short-grain brown
   rice
50 ml (2 fl oz) Marsala
1.2 litres (2 pints) vegetable stock
125 g (4 oz) asparagus tips,
   chopped
salt and pepper
finely grated Parmesan cheese,
   to serve (optional)

1 Drain the porcini, reserving the soaking liquid, then squeeze dry and roughly chop.

2 Heat the butter and oil in a large, flameproof casserole over a low heat, add the shallots and leek and fry gently for 8 minutes or until softened. Add the garlic and fry for a further 2 minutes. Stir the rice into the pan and cook for 1–2 minutes, then pour over the Marsala and bubble, stirring continuously, until evaporated.

3 Mix in the mushrooms, reserved soaking liquid and stock, stir well and bring to the boil. Season to taste with salt and pepper, cover and place in a preheated oven, 180°C (350°F), Gas Mark 4, for 45 minutes, stirring occasionally.

4 Add the asparagus and stir well. Return to the oven for a further 15 minutes or until the rice is tender and most of the liquid has been absorbed. Remove from the oven and leave to stand for 2–3 minutes. Spoon the risotto into serving bowls and sprinkle with the grated Parmesan, if liked.

Tip
Unlike most risottos, this baked version is very entertaining-friendly as you can pop it in the oven and it needs stirring only every now and then.

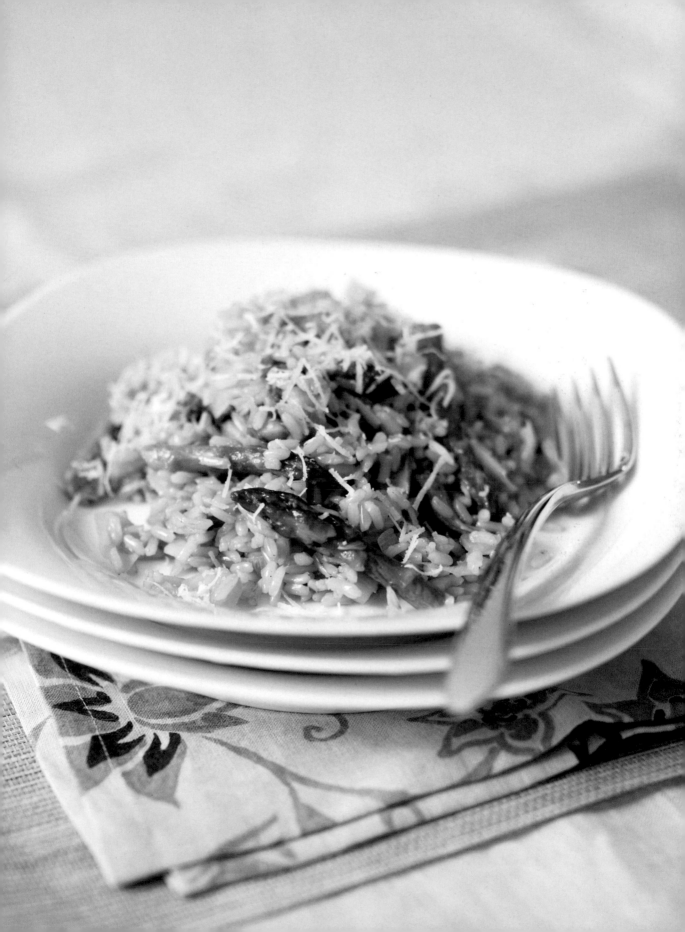

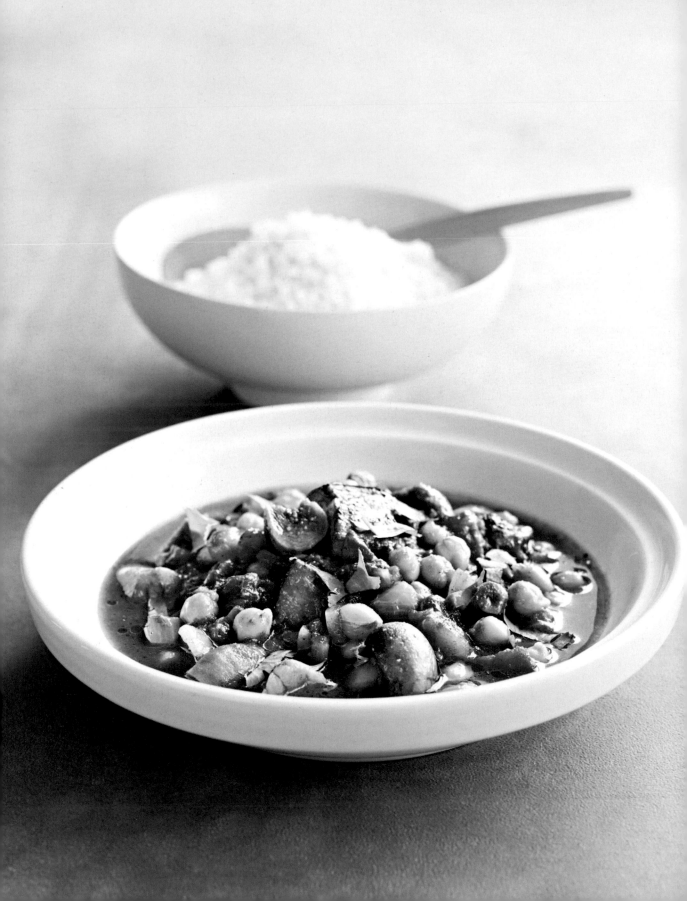

saffron-scented vegetable tagine

serves 4
prep + cook time 1 hour

100 ml (3½ fl oz) sunflower oil
1 large onion, finely chopped
2 garlic cloves, finely chopped
2 teaspoons ground coriander
2 teaspoons ground cumin
2 teaspoons ground cinnamon
400 g (13 oz) can chickpeas,
    drained
400 g (13 oz) can chopped
    tomatoes
600 ml (1 pint) vegetable stock
¼ teaspoon saffron threads
1 large aubergine, chopped
250 g (8 oz) button mushrooms,
    halved if large
100 g (3½ oz) dried figs, chopped
2 tablespoons chopped coriander
salt and pepper

1 Heat 2 tablespoons of the oil in a frying pan over a medium heat, add the onion, garlic and spices and cook, stirring frequently, for 5 minutes or until golden. Using a slotted spoon, transfer to a saucepan and add the chickpeas, tomatoes, stock and saffron. Season with salt and pepper.

2 Heat the remaining oil in the frying pan over a high heat, add the aubergine and cook, stirring frequently, for 5 minutes or until browned. Add to the stew and bring to the boil, then reduce the heat, cover and simmer gently for 20 minutes.

3 Stir in the mushrooms and figs and simmer gently, uncovered, for a further 20 minutes. Stir in the chopped coriander and season to taste. Serve with steamed wholewheat couscous.

Tip
Saffron threads are the dried stamens from a particular type of crocus and are used to give curries, rice dishes and desserts a musky fragrance and golden colour.

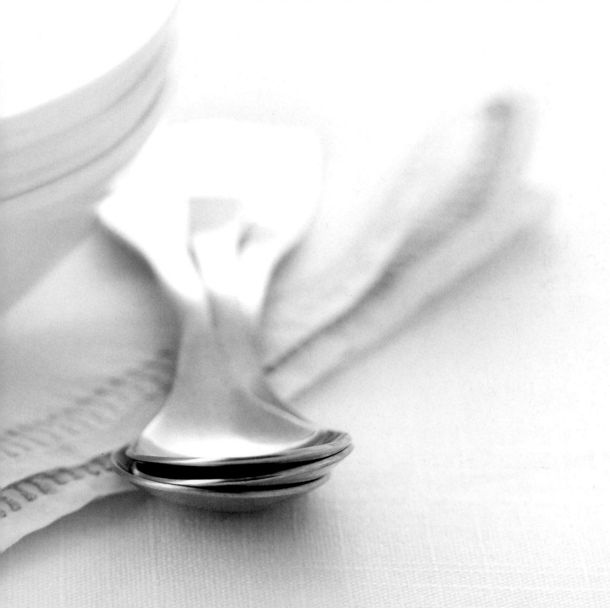

healthy
desserts

fresh berries with crunchy oats

serves 4
prep + cook time 30 minutes

500 g (1 lb) mixed berries, such
    as black and redcurrants,
    blueberries, strawberries,
    raspberries and blackberries
1 teaspoon orange blossom water
¼ teaspoon mixed spice
1–2 tablespoons soft dark brown
    sugar (optional)
200 g (7 oz) crunchy oat cereal,
    such as almond and raisin

1 Preheat the oven to 180°C (350°F), Gas Mark 4. Wash and hull the fresh berries, if necessary.

2 Place the berries in a large bowl with the orange blossom water, mixed spice and sugar, if using, and toss until well combined. Tip the coated fruits into an ovenproof dish, then sprinkle the oat cereal over the fruits, pressing down to flatten.

3 Bake in the oven for 18–20 minutes until golden and crisp, then remove from the oven and serve immediately.

Tip
Bright, delicious and low in fat, berries are packed with health-boosting antioxidants. You can vary the berries you use in this winter dessert.

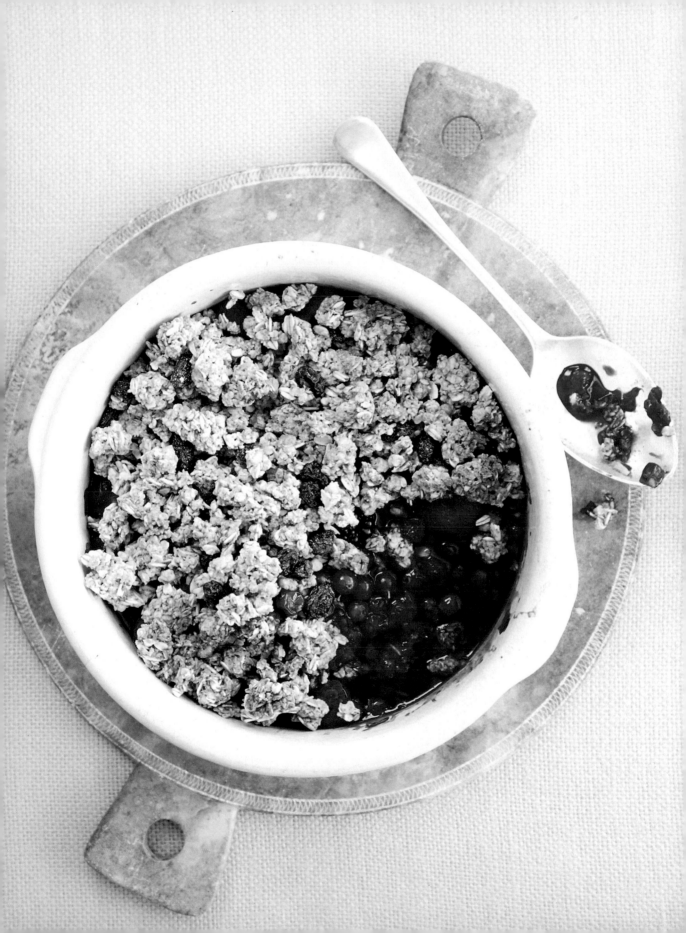

grilled nectarines with mint vanilla cream

serves 4
prep + cook time 17–18 minutes

4 nectarines, halved and stoned
pinch of ground cinnamon
1 tablespoon clear honey
grated rind and juice of 1 orange

to serve
4 tablespoons reduced-fat crème
   fraîche
150 g (5 oz) natural yogurt
1 tablespoon chopped mint
few drops of vanilla extract

1 Place the nectarines on a grill pan, cut side up. Mix together the cinnamon, honey and orange rind and juice, and drizzle over the nectarines.
2 Place the nectarines under a preheated hot grill and cook for 7–8 minutes until golden, basting occasionally with the juices.
3 Mix together the crème fraîche, yogurt, mint and vanilla extract and serve with the nectarines.

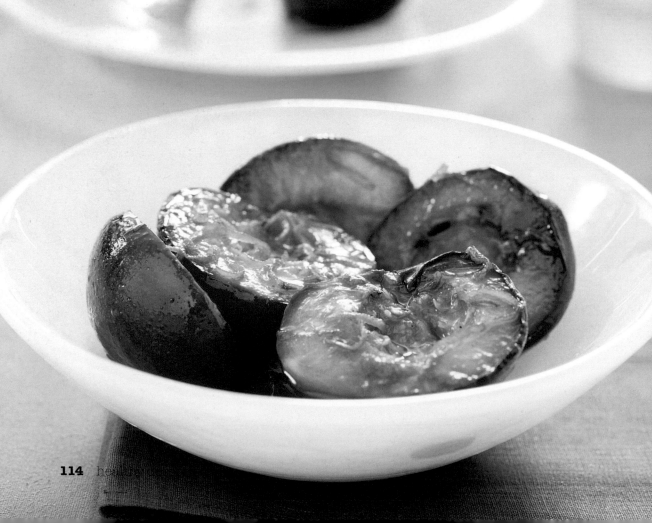

griddled pineapple & ginger

serves 4
prep + cook time 10 minutes

2 tablespoons icing sugar
1 teaspoon ground ginger
1 pineapple, peeled and cut into
  2.5 cm (1 inch) thick rounds
4 tablespoons reduced-fat
  fromage frais, to serve

1 Heat a griddle or a heavy-based frying pan until hot.
2 Mix together the icing sugar and ginger and sprinkle over both sides of the pineapple rings. Place the pineapple on the griddle and cook for 1–2 minutes on each side until golden.
3 Serve the pineapple hot with the fromage frais.

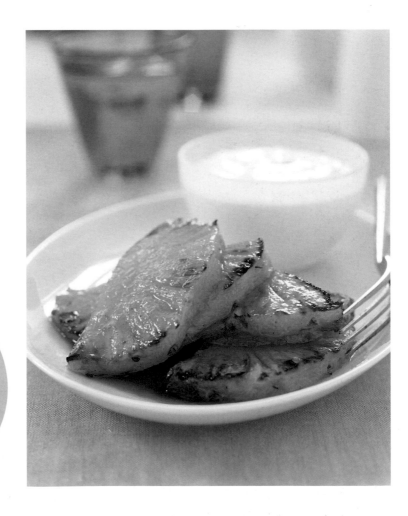

Tip
Pineapple contains bromelain, an enzyme which breaks down protein.

individual lime & raspberry cheesecakes

serves 4
prep time 10 minutes

6 ginger biscuits, lightly crushed
200 g (7 oz) reduced-fat cream
   cheese
200 g (7 oz) reduced-fat fromage
   frais
few drops of vanilla extract
1 tablespoon caster sugar
grated rind and juice of 1 lime
125 g (4 oz) raspberries
lime wedges, to garnish

1 Divide the biscuits between 4 small glasses.
2 In a bowl, mix together the cream cheese, fromage frais, vanilla extract, sugar, and lime rind and juice.
3 Spoon the mixture on to the biscuits, then top with the raspberries. Serve immediately garnished with a lime wedge.

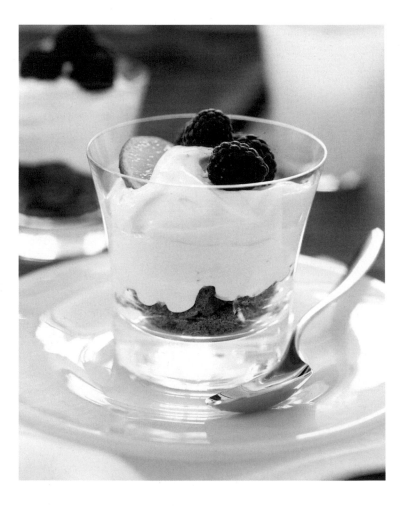

Tip
Choose very fresh raspberries as they have a higher antioxidant content and are more nutritious.

mango & passion fruit trifles

serves 4
prep time 10 minutes

4 sponge fingers
150 g (5 oz) reduced-fat Greek
    yogurt
200 g (7 oz) reduced-fat fromage
    frais
4 passion fruit
1 mango, peeled, stoned and
    diced

1 Break each biscuit into 4 pieces and arrange them in 4 glasses.
2 Mix together the yogurt and crème fraîche. Remove the seedy pulp from the passion fruit and set aside.
3 Spoon a little passion fruit pulp over the biscuits and then add about half of the mango pieces.
4 Pour about half the crème fraîche mix over the fruit and top with the remaining mango.
5 Top with the remaining crème fraîche mix and arrange the rest of the passion fruit on top. Refrigerate for up to 1 hour or serve immediately.

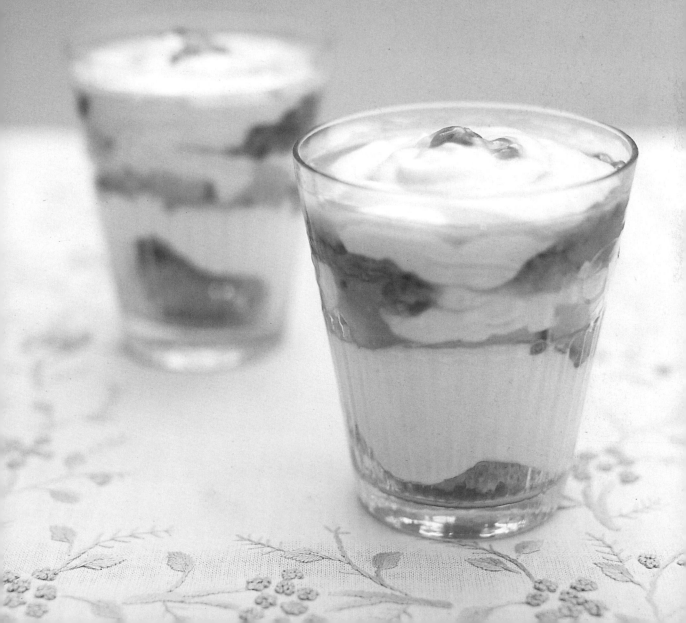

poached apricots with orange flower water & pistachios

serves 4
prep time 10 minutes

400 g (13 oz) ready-to-eat
   semi-dried apricots
350 ml (12 fl oz) apple and
   elderflower juice
2 tablespoons orange flower water
½ teaspoon ground cinnamon
2 tablespoons clear honey
75 g (3 oz) shelled unsalted
   pistachios, crushed, to serve

1 Put the apricots in a pan with the apple and elderflower juice, orange flower water, cinnamon and honey and bring to a gentle boil over a medium-high heat. Reduce the heat and simmer for 2–3 minutes until fragrant.
2 Pour the apricots and juices into a large bowl and set aside to cool slightly.
3 Scatter with pistachios and serve.

Tip
Orange flower water adds a distinctive citrus-floral flavour to this refreshing Moroccan dessert. You'll find it in the baking aisle of most supermarkets.

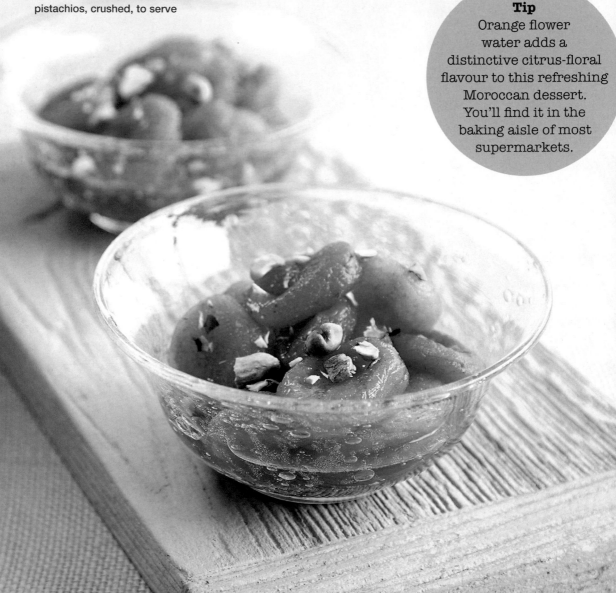

passion fruit panna cotta

serves 4
prep time 20 minutes + setting time

2 gelatine leaves
8 passion fruit
200 g (7 oz) reduced-fat fromage
  frais
125 g (4 oz) reduced-fat Greek
  yogurt
1 teaspoon caster sugar
vanilla pod, split

1 Soften the gelatine leaves in cold water. Halve the passion fruit and remove the seeds, working over a bowl to catch as much juice as you can. Reserve the seeds for decoration.
2 Combine the crème fraîche, yogurt and passion fruit juice.
3 Put 100 ml (3½ fl oz) water in a small saucepan, add the sugar and the seeds from the vanilla pod and heat gently, stirring until the sugar has dissolved. Drain the gelatine and add to the pan. Stir until dissolved, then leave to cool to room temperature.
4 Mix the gelatine mixture into the crème fraîche, then pour into 4 ramekins or moulds. Refrigerate for 6 hours or until set.
5 Turn the panna cotta out of their moulds by briefly immersing each ramekin in very hot water. Spoon over the reserved seeds to decorate.

For coffee panna cotta, substitute 2 teaspoons strong coffee for the passion fruit and continue as for the recipe above. Decorate each panna cotta with chocolate coffee beans, if you like.

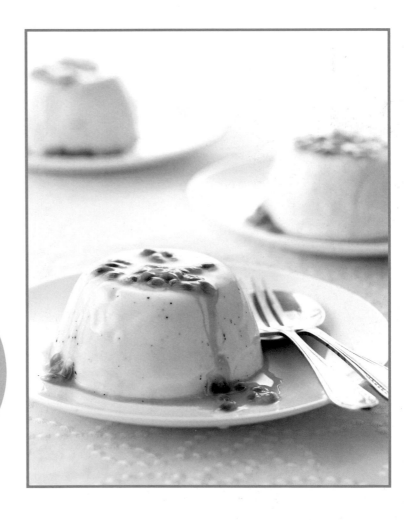

mango, cardamom & mint fools

serves 6
prep time 20 minutes + chilling time

625 g (1¼ lb) reduced-fat Greek yogurt, chilled
5 green cardamom pods, seeds finely crushed
2 tablespoons icing sugar
grated rind and juice of 1 lime
200 ml (7 fl oz) canned mango purée
2 tablespoons chopped mint

to decorate
chopped mango
mint sprigs

1 Place the yogurt, crushed cardamom, icing sugar, lime rind and juice in a large bowl and slowly whisk together with a hand-held electric whisk for 1–2 minutes.
2 Whisk in the mango pureé until combined, then stir in the mint. Spoon into 6 glasses and chill for 10 minutes.
3 Serve decorated with chopped mango and a mint sprig.

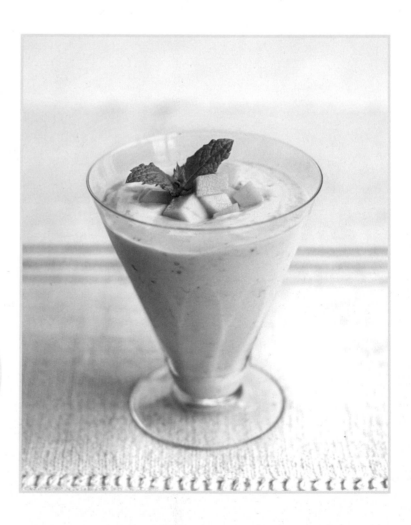

Tip
This low-fat fool is a perfect choice to end a summer meal. For a more decadent version, use whipped double cream instead of the yogurt.

balsamic & black pepper strawberries

serves 4
prep time 10 minutes

500g (1 lb) strawberries, hulled
    and halved
2 tablespoons balsamic vinegar
1 teaspoon freshly ground
black pepper

1 Place the strawberries in a bowl and pour over the vinegar.
2 Stir well, to incorporate the flavours, then add the black pepper to taste. Serve immediately.

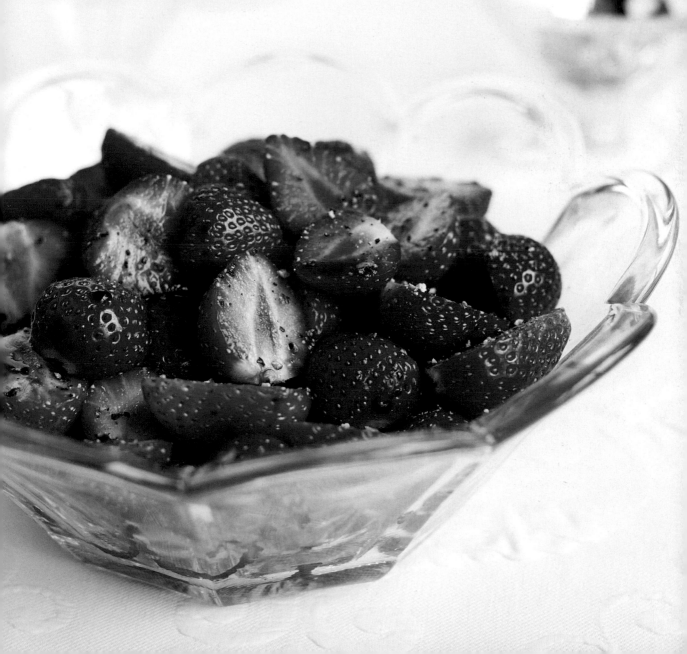

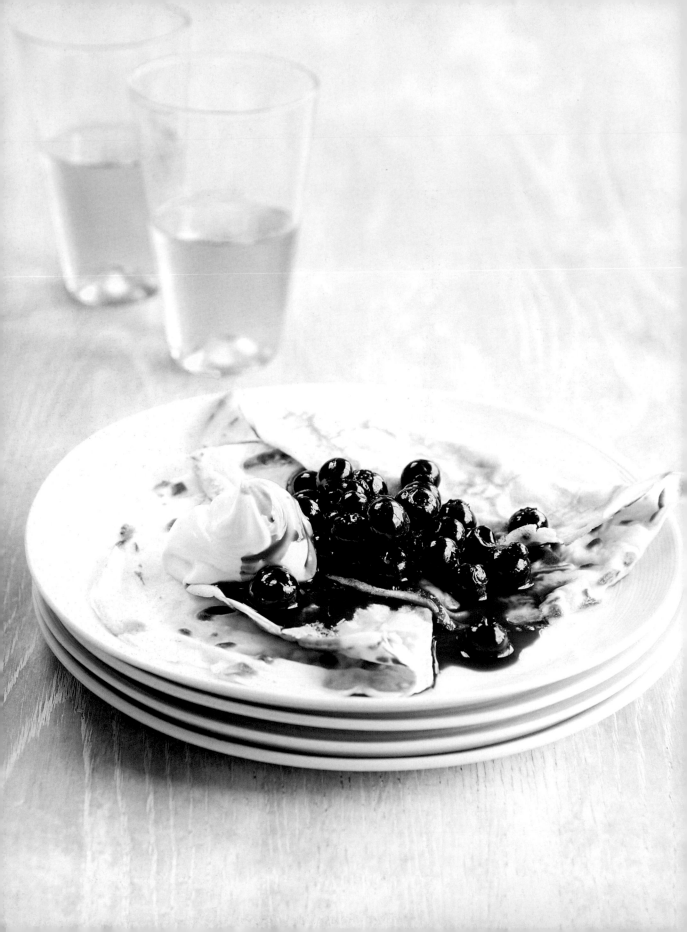

pancakes with vanilla blueberries

serves 4
prep time 30 minutes

250 g (8 oz) blueberries
2 tablespoons freshly squeezed
   orange juice
1–2 tablespoons vanilla sugar,
   to taste
vegetable oil, for greasing
4 tablespoons reduced-fat crème
   fraîche, to serve (optional)

pancake mix
125 g (4 oz) plain flour
1 egg
300 ml (½ pint) skimmed milk

1 Put the pancake ingredients in a blender and process until smooth. Leave to rest for 10 minutes.
2 Meanwhile, place the blueberries, orange juice and vanilla sugar, to taste, in a small saucepan over a low heat and warm gently until the blueberries begin to burst. Remove from the heat and set aside to cool slightly.
3 Heat a small, nonstick pancake pan or small frying pan over a medium heat and grease the surface lightly with a little vegetable oil. Pour a little batter into the pan and swirl to coat thinly; the mixture should make 8 pancakes in total. Cook gently for 2 minutes or until golden underneath, then flip over the pancake and cook the other side for about 30 seconds. Slide on to a plate, cover with a piece of baking parchment and repeat the process to make the remaining pancakes.
4 To serve, fold 2 pancakes on to each serving plate and spoon over the warm vanilla blueberries. Serve with a dollop of half-fat crème fraîche, if desired.

Tip
To make vanilla sugar, slice a vanilla pod in two lengthways, place in an airtight container and cover with 100 g caster sugar. Seal and leave for 24 hours and up to 2 weeks for the sugar to absorb the vanilla.

summer fruit compote

serves 2
prep time 10 minutes + chilling time

250 g (8 oz) mixed summer fruit,
    such as raspberries, blueberries
    and strawberries, thawed if
    frozen
finely grated rind and juice of
    1 large orange
1 tablespoon redcurrant jelly
250 g (8 oz) reduced-fat Greek
    yogurt, to serve

1 Put the fruit, orange rind and juice and redcurrant jelly in a large saucepan. Cover and cook gently for 5 minutes or until the juices flow and the fruit is softened.

2 Remove the pan from the heat and set aside. When the fruit is cool, chill it and serve with yogurt.

Tip
Blueberries are full of antioxidants and research suggests that they are good for heart and bones.

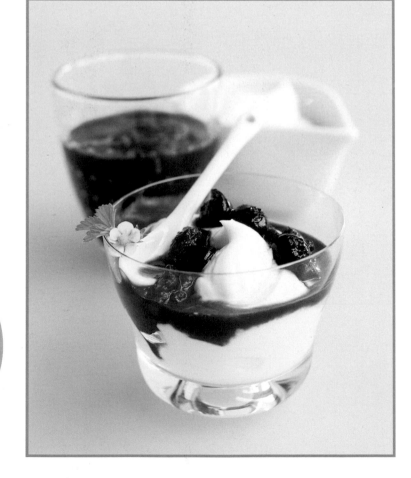

frozen berry yogurt ice cream

serves 4
prep time 10 minute

400 g (13 oz) frozen mixed summer
    berries, such as raspberries,
    blueberries and blackberries
250 g (8 oz) reduced-fat Greek
    yogurt
2 tablespoons icing sugar
wafers, to serve (optional)

1 Place half the berries, the yogurt and icing sugar in a food
processor or blender and blend until fairly smooth and the berries have
broken up.
2 Add the rest of the berries and pulse until they are slightly broken
up but some texture remains. Place scoops of the yogurt ice cream
into bowls and serve immediately with wafers, if liked.

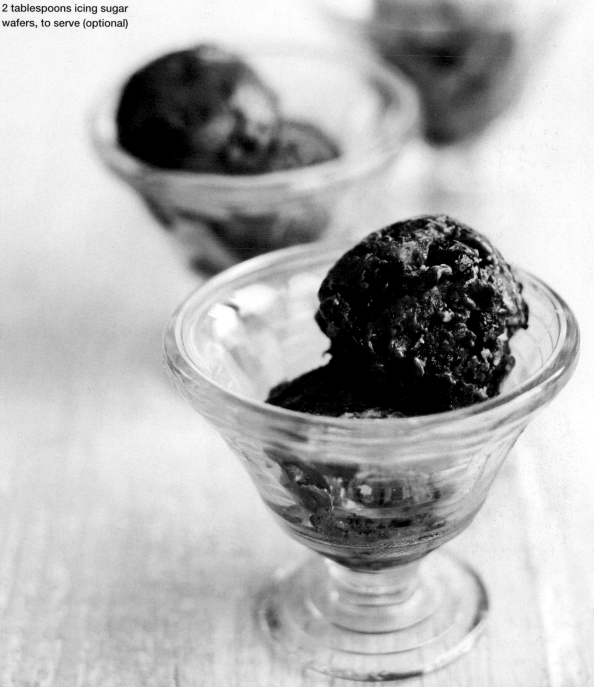

index

Acknowledgements
578foot/Shutterstock 2–3.
Special photography © Octopus Publishing Group/
Stephen Conroy 95.
Will Heap 43, 63, 70, 83, 96, 99, 120, 121, 125.
Jeremy Hopley 1, 50, 53.
William Lingwood 45.
David Munns 47, 89, 93.
Lis Parsons 5, 15, 31, 39, 60–61, 64, 87, 88, 110–111, 113, 117, 118, 119, 122, 124.
Photodisc 8 (bottom).
William Reveall 6, 8 (top), 9, 10, 16, 17, 22, 23, 24, 26, 27, 29, 30, 32, 34, 35, 40, 51, 54,
    55, 57, 58, 59, 65, 68, 69, 72, 73, 80, 81, 100, 114, 115, 116.
Craig Robertson 41, 79, 104, 105.
Gareth Sambidge 11, 44.
William Shaw 19, 20, 46, 48, 66, 75, 76, 77, 84–85, 90, 101, 102, 107, 108.
Ian Wallace 12–13, 36–37, 95.